Interpersonal Communication and Psychology for Health Care Professionals:
Theory and Practice

Dev. M. Rungapadiachy

MSc (Applied Psychology), BSc (Hons)
Nursing Studies, DPSN, Cert Ed., FETC, RMN, RGN
Lecturer in (psychology and interpersonal communication)
School of Health Care Studies
University of Leeds

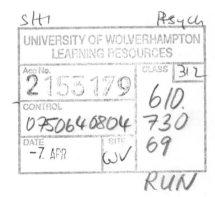

BUTTERWORTH
HEINEMANN

OXFORD   AUCKLAND   BOSTON   JOHANNESBURG   MELBOURNE   NEW DELHI

Butterworth-Heinemann
Linacre House, Jordan Hill, Oxford OX2 8DP
225 Wildwood Avenue, Woburn, MA 01801-2041
A division of Reed Educational and Professional Publishing Ltd

A member of the Reed Elsevier plc group

First published 1999

© Dev. M. Rungapadiachy 1999

British Library Cataloguing in Publication Data
A catalogue record for this book is available from the British Library

Library of Congress Cataloguing in Publication Data
A catalogue record for this book is available from the Library of Congress

ISBN 0 7506 4080 4

Composition and design by Scribe Design Gillingham, Kent
Printed and bound in Great Britain

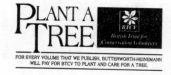

Contents

Preface

Defined as a scientific study of human behaviour, psychology can also be seen as the 'raison d'être' of interpersonal communication. Interpersonal communication signifies person to person (or persons) interaction. Psychology therefore attempts to offer possible rationales for the way people interact with one another and behave in general. For example, why am I writing this book? From a psychological point of view the answer rests in my motivation. I was motivated by such questions as 'Are interpersonal skills and psychology different?' 'Should they be grouped and taught as one theme?' My position has always been clear in that both psychology and interpersonal skills can indeed be taught as one theme. Educationalists however, have to ensure that students become aware of the fact that psychology underpins interpersonal skills. Many of the explanations of human behaviour rest in the realm of psychology. Whilst psychology can be taught without the mere mention of interpersonal communication, the same cannot be said for the facilitation of the latter. Teaching or facilitating interpersonal skills without some of its underlying psychological principles would be like teaching human biology without mentioning the human body. Interpersonal communication is inextricably linked with psychology and as such they should be taught in tandem, especially as far as health care delivery is concerned. In most cases people behave differently when well, as compared to when they become ill. The rationales for such behaviour can be found in the person's intrapersonal dynamics.

This provided me with the three themes to focus on and these are intrapersonal, interpersonal and those interpersonal skills that are prerequisites for health care professionals. These elements became the backbone of the book, having said that some of the theories make it such that these clear-cut divisions became too confusing to maintain. Most of the theories contain the two dimensions of intra- and interpersonal elements. This would have meant a great deal of cross referencing. Reviewers and critics would have had a field day, to say that this book is about interpersonal communication, psychology and health care. Common sense prevailed and the structure offered is such that there are elements of intra- and interpersonal dynamics in both, Section I and Section II. The emphasis throughout is on the concept of self-awareness as an enhancer of care delivery. My overall sentiment is that the foundation for caring or helping is firmly grounded in self-awareness. Knowing one's strengths, weaknesses, likes and dislikes, attitudes and values, is one of the ways of safeguarding clients' or patients' health and well-being. Similarly reflection is the very essence of self-awareness and the book offers opportunities for reflecting on self as a means to enhancing self-awareness. Current health care philosophies stress the need to be reflective in practice, thus ensuring a better quality of care. To this end activities are included to encourage readers' reflective interaction. Appropriately enough the opening chapter discusses the concept of self-awareness and the closing chapter considers reflection.

Acknowledgements

I would agree with those numerous authors who have remarked that writing a book is a lonely venture. I must add, however, that in this case the conception and birth of my book kept me occupied whilst the loneliness was endured and experienced by those who are most precious to me, my wife Devi and my two children Jason and Darren. Having said that I have attempted to involve them as much as possible, the end-product has thus meant a true family venture. I express my sincere thanks to Devi, for freeing me from the burden of domestic responsibilities and for still being my dear friend and wife; to Jason, for the 12 cute little meerkats which add some humour to Heron's concept of intervention, for the faces of emotion and for putting up with my constant harassment until the drawings were complete; and to Darren, for your patience, understanding and skills shown in all those remaining illustrations. My admiration also to you Darren, for taming my beastly computer which was my master but became your slave.

I would also like to thank Abdul Kapdi and Mike Thornton for their expert help and advice with computer technology, Jean Allison and Ern Hall for their continuous support and understanding throughout this venture, and last but not least, my friend, counsellor, supervisor, and confidante, Anne Lawton, who listened when I needed to ventilate.

My warm and sincere thanks to Helen Reece, your reassurance, comfort and help made the journey less arduous.

A sincere thank you to all those students whose evaluations of some of the chapters were very much appreciated, as for copies of the book, well you have to buy them, no free copies I'm afraid.

Dev. M. Rungapadiachy, 1998

Introduction

Communication a central core to health care delivery

Communication is now recognised as an essential part of health care delivery. From a medical point of view Myerscough (1992, p.2) argues, 'the need to acquire the necessary professional knowledge, skills, and attitudes. . . to learn the scientific basis from which the art of competent communication is derived. . . has been recognised'. From a nursing perspective, communication in the form of interpersonal skills training has become part and parcel of the educational package. Other health care disciplines such as radiography, radiotherapy, dental nursing and so on, have included communication as part of the teaching programme. Over the past 30 years, a number of surveys (Cartwright, 1964; Raphael, 1969; Skeet, 1970) have shown that patients tend to be more critical about poor communication between staff and patients than about any other aspect of their hospital experience. Let's face it, if anyone of us is kept in the dark as to what is really happening to us, wouldn't we go berserk? One could argue therefore that communication is central to care delivery, in whatever capacity or health care discipline one happens to be. This implies that good communication leads to better and higher standards of care. To be fair I have to admit that I am not telling you something that you do not already know. In fact most of the literature and books on the subject of communication emphasise this very point. Numerous authors have also written extensively on the skills one needs to have in order to be a better communicator. So why write another book, when everything, well almost everything, has been said before? Am I just jumping on the bandwagon to write for the sake of academic credibility? What really have I to offer?

Well, this may not be such a difficult question to answer. My years of experience as both a clinician and an educationalist have led me to believe that the words 'interpersonal skills' and 'communication' are seen as a series of exercises or 'games', which may be fun but frightening and their relevance is questioned by those who have an aversion to experiential learning activities, (the concept of experiential learning is discussed later) including both tutors and students. I have thought long and hard as to why some students (and tutors) perceive interpersonal skills training in particular as games. Could this have any bearing on the way we (by 'we' I include myself) portray these. Of course most of us will swear that we do our best to make the training as interactive and interesting as we possibly can. So where exactly does the problem lie? My general belief is that there are at least three problems in either the way we conduct our educational process or how we write on the subject.

Intra- and interpersonal dimensions of self

Firstly, it may well be that some of the structured exercises are not followed by the underpinning theory or theories. I do appreciate that this may be for various reasons and one which easily springs to mind is the shortage of time. A limited number of hours are allotted to interpersonal skills and psychology in most health care syllabi. This in itself may be a reflection on how important or unimportant interpersonal skills and psychology are perceived to be.

Secondly, it can be said that interpersonal communication focuses on the interaction between individuals and although there is an abundance of literature on the subject, nevertheless very few, if any, emphasise the intrapersonal elements which are the driving forces of interpersonal communication. 'A great part of human communication is emotional communication, involving minute signals of affect, attention, approach and avoidance, dominance and submission, that convey information of central importance to human social organisation' (Buck, 1984, p.3). This is more than non-verbal communication. This involves much deeper intrapersonal issues. Condon (1980, p.63) argues, 'communication is not just a process of "bits" of information travelling between people. It is as much an overreaching domain of trust and distrust, the multitudinous and subtle ways by which people love and hate, praise and blame, accept and reject themselves as well as others. As such they affect the inner being of others, there to aid or hinder, with greater or lesser consequences on that inner life.' There is little doubt that the key to understanding human behaviours rests within oneself. The implication is that it is only by getting to know oneself that one stands a chance to know and to communicate with others. When looking at any interaction therefore both the intra- and the interpersonal aspects of people should be explored. Let us say for the sake

Figure i

The visible and invisible dimensions of 'Me'

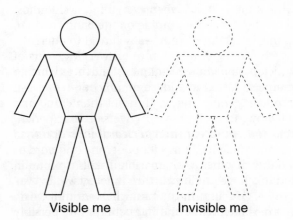

Visible me   Invisible me

of argument that each one of us can be viewed from two dimensions, and these are internal and external. I will call these invisible and visible 'me' respectively. Figure i shows a graphic display of the aspects of self.

The factors that actually characterise and guide the invisible 'me' are past experiences from previous encounters. By the very nature of one's conception, birth, growth and development, self has never existed alone. Self is always influenced by significant others. For this reason therefore one could argue that self can never be studied from what Laing *et al.* (1966, p.3) called an egoistic standpoint.

Past experience as a foundation for future encounter

'Some philosophers, some psychologists, and more sociologists have recognised the significance of the fact that social life is not made up of a myriad I's and Me's only, but of you, he, she, we and them, also and that the experience of you or he or them or us may indeed be as primary and compelling (or more so) as the experience of "me".' Each and every encounter has as its very foundation 'Past Experiences'. In any interaction therefore what really happens can be seen in Figure ii.

Past experience and present encounter

Figure ii
Interactions between the two components of self and those of other (s)

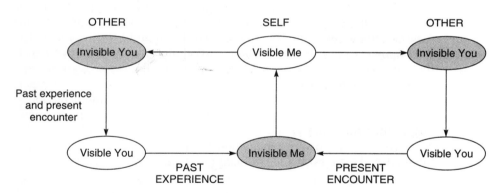

Each new encounter becomes a building block for past experiences which, in turn, energise future encounters (see Figure iii).

New encounters as building blocks for past experiences

Intrapersonal dynamics as the source of interpersonal interactions

Before self can communicate with other, the 'invisible me' has to feed information to the 'visible me'. The 'visible me' then interacts with the 'invisible you' first, the 'invisible you' in turn communicates with the 'visible you'. From this perspective therefore the starting point of any person

Figure iii

Past experiences as building blocks for future encounters

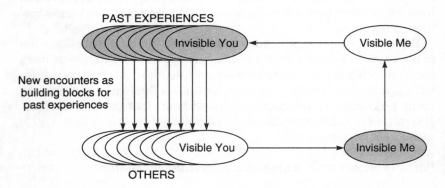

to person interaction has to be with one's intrapersonal dynamics, and these are clearly influenced by one's past experiences. So why look at the 'visible' and 'invisible me' communicating with the 'visible' and 'invisible you', when what we should be doing is considering how we got to be who we are at the here and now. The answer for this the author believes rests in the concept of intrapersonal dynamics. Equipped with this knowledge, one can then move on to new encounters with others.

Thirdly, self-awareness is seen as important to care delivery but only a handful of writers have attempted to link the theory of self-awareness to its applications to clinical practice. How students' concepts of their own self-awareness can enhance care delivery is left for them to fathom out. Although the ideas of self-discovery and self-direction are quite attractive, nevertheless one has to admit that there is a limit to how much one can learn through this process.

What this book offers

This book attempts to deal with those three issues which have been raised. Its main theme is interpersonal communication as applied to health care delivery. Having said that the author would argue that the theories which underpin interpersonal communication lie in psychology. The discipline of psychology attempts to explain why people think, feel and act as they do. Each individual would seem to function from his or her own internal frame of reference. It is clear therefore that a knowledge of the various perspectives in psychology would help to enhance one's understanding of people's behaviour. This book provides the opportunity to explore those 'classic' psychological perspectives which offer their particular explanations of human behaviour, these include psychoanalytical, behavioural, social learning, cognitive, humanistic, psychosocial, and interpersonal perspectives. Some aspects of social psychology which have a direct influence on health care delivery are also discussed, these are in the shape of attitudes, values, beliefs, prejudice, stereotype, discrimination, obedience, conformity, compliance and learned helplessness. Both emotion and stress are elements which affect one's interaction with the environment, and as such they cannot be ignored. A chapter is therefore dedicated to each of these concepts.

Communication is explored from two perspectives and these are: communication at a general level and communication at a therapeutic level. The therapeutic level of communication deals with such concepts as listening, attending, responding, trust, disclosure, feedback, assertiveness, Heron's six-category intervention analysis and transactional analysis. Two models of helping are also explored and they are that of Egan (1975) and that of Brammer (1988).

Who this book is for and the level it is aimed at

The whole sentiment of this book is focused around the concept of helping. Any behaviour or activity which seeks to enhance growth, development and personal autonomy on the part of the patients/clients falls under the realm of helping. Any professional group or discipline, whose sole purpose is to offer help to patients/clients is identified as health care professionals. This includes doctors, nurses, psychologists, counsellors, psychotherapists, radiographers, radiotherapists, occupational therapists, audiologists, dental nurses, physiotherapists, midwives, health visitors, social workers, and so on. If you are a student in any one of these disciplines, and your interest is in communication and helping, then this book is for you. I am aware that there are books on both interpersonal communication and psychology, but each subject so far is presented separately. You could pick up a book on interpersonal communication and you will find the focus restricted to that particular subject. Similarly a book on psychology will offer you a specific focus or a focus in general. I plan to offer an in-depth insight of the theory of interpersonal communication and some of its skills, together with some relevant aspects of psychology. The book should essentially offer enough information to see you through any course up to and possibly above graduate level, depending on your chosen discipline. What I propose to do is to demonstrate clearly how one's knowledge of oneself can benefit both oneself and those under one's care.

Organisation of the book

The contents are classified into three main themes and these are discussed in three sections.

Section I – Intrapersonal dynamics and self-awareness

The emphasis of Chapter 1 is on issues related to self-awareness, its tri-components and different layers. Reflection on one's internal dynamics is a common theme throughout. One could say that the very root of self-awareness rests in Freud's psychoanalytical theory of personality development. Chapter 2 describes the basic tenet of psychoanalytical theory. Luft and Ingham's (1955) Johari Window is described in an attempt to show the four facets (open, blind, hidden and unknown) of self. Chapter 3 explores Eric Berne's (1964) transactional analysis and its significance to health care delivery. Attempts are made to explain how a knowledge of transactional analysis can enhance health care delivery. Chapter 4 offers some of Piaget's (1952) thoughts on cognitive development. The emphasis is on schema formation and stages of cognitive development. The works of

Tolman (1958) and Kohler (1925) are filtered through and Kohlberg's (1981) notion of moral development is described. Chapter 5 emphasises certain key features of perception where Snyder's (1974) notion of self-monitoring is introduced. Chapter 6 explores the humanistic's concept of behaviour, the works of both Rogers (1951) and Maslow (1954) are discussed. Chapter 7 delves into the dynamics of emotion and in particular anger. Some of the theories of anger are explained and its relevance to health care delivery is highlighted. Chapter 8 reviews some aspects of social psychology in the form of attitudes and prejudices on behaviour. Stockwell's (1984) notion of the unpopular patient concludes Section I.

Section II – Interpersonal behaviour and self-awareness

This section addresses those observable behaviours and the underpinning theories as to why one behaves the way one does. Having said that it is well known that all theories have their own strengths and weaknesses, the approach adopted here is a non-evaluative one. As such therefore it is not intended to critique any of the theories discussed in this book. The first two chapters of Section II (Chapters 9 and 10) offer an insight into Sullivan's (1953) interpersonal and Erikson's (1963) psychosocial theories respectively. Chapter 11 stresses the notion of learning as possible explanations of behaviour. The emphasis is on Watson's (1930) and Pavlov's (1927) classical conditioning, Skinner's (1974) operant conditioning and Bandura's (1974) social learning. Chapter 12 focuses on stress and behaviour. Selye's (1976) biological, Holmes and Rahe's (1967) life events, Lazarus and Folkman's (1984) cognitive appraisal and Cox's (1978) transactional models of stress are explained. The chapter also offers a brief insight into the notion of anxiety and its implication for communication. Chapter 13 reviews other aspects of social psychology and in particular obedience, conformity and compliance. The work of Milgram (1974), Asch (1952), Hofling *et al.* (1966) and Zimbardo (1992) are discussed. Also included is Seligman's (1975) concept of learned helplessness and its implication to health care delivery. Chapter 14 involves group formation and dynamics, roles, leadership and leadership styles in the form of autocratic, democratic and laissez-faire. Chapter 15 unravels the nature and dynamics of interpersonal conflict and ways of dealing with it. Conflict resolution is dependent on effective interpersonal skills which form the very essence of Section III.

Section III – Interpersonal skills and practice

This section explores some of the skills of interpersonal communication. The introduction to this section summarises the core skills of communication in the form of a model. Chapter 16 examines the various dimensions of communication, these include proxemics, territoriality, gaze, touch and silence. Chapter 17 explains some of the micro-skills of communication and these fall in the domain of listening, attending and responding, the main focus is on therapeutic listening. The essence of a therapeutic relationship is discussed in Chapter 18 in the form of trust, disclosure and feedback. Johari Window is revisited in an attempt to explain how trust, disclosure and feedback can lead to a greater sense of awareness and hence enhancing the rapport between helper and client/patient. Chapter 19 centres around the concept of assertive behaviour and its effect on care delivery. Assertiveness is discussed in relation to submissiveness and aggressiveness, the latter two are seen as non-therapeutic to clients/patients. The concept of therapeutic care forms the basis of Chapter 20 and explores Heron's six-category intervention analysis. This chapter stresses those non-therapeutic activities such as degenerative and perverted interventions in order to show the vulnerability of clients/patients. Heron's therapeutic interventions are discussed and the skills involved are highlighted. Chapter 21 offers a brief overview of Egan's (1975) and Brammer's (1988) models of helping. Some of the focus is on: the strategies of helping, the characteristics of a helper, and the different barriers to helping. Chapter 22 reflects on some of the main issues of the previous chapters and attempts to show how self-awareness can in fact enhance health care delivery.

Experiential exercises are included to help the reader relate to the concepts under discussion. The general flavour is a mixture of theory, self-exploration, and reflection from these exercises. Reflection captures the essence of pausing and looking back at any issue which has emerged during one's life experiences. The concept of self-exploration may be old, nevertheless the therapeutic use of self in care delivery is very much in its infancy. Reflective caring is now the way forward, this therefore is one of the reasons why reflection underpins the philosophy of this book. O'Connor and Seymour's (1990) model of learning is adapted to stress the importance of reflection in clinical practice.

The process of learning

Imagine you want to learn how to drive a car. At this point in time one would say that 'you know that you don't know how to drive a car'. O'Connor and Seymour call this, 'The State of Conscious Incompetence'. Your learning process would therefore start with you undergoing driving instructions from a competent driver.

State of conscious incompetence

At some point your instructor will evaluate your skills and accordingly, will decide that you should apply for your test. Meanwhile you carry on with your practice until you take your test. You realise by this time that you know how to drive a car. You take your test and at the end of the test you hear the much welcome words 'I am pleased to tell you that you have passed, congratulations'. All the doubts that you may have had before your test disappear. You are now at the learning stage of 'You know that you know', this is known as 'The State of Conscious Competence'. Your red L plate goes in the bin and is replaced by a green one. You are now gradually getting increasingly confident about your driving and with the passage of time most of what you have learnt becomes second nature to you.

State of conscious competence

State of unconscious competence

You now drive your car without having to think about it. You in fact enter the stage of not knowing that you know, this is translated as 'The State of Unconscious Competence'. What really happens when you function at the state of unconscious competence is that along the way you would have collected bad habits, through taking short cuts and such like behaviours. Eventually your competency is in doubt but sadly you are the last one to know. You reach the stage of 'You don't know that you don't know,' this is translated as 'The State of Unconscious Incompetence'. As far as your driving skills are concerned, you are now worse off than you were when you first started your lessons, at least then you knew that you did not know. Here, however, you don't even know that you don't know. Translating this into a health care scenario one can imagine the damage one can cause purely as a result of lack of conscious awareness. The concept of reflection goes some way to preventing anyone reaching the states of unconscious competence and unconscious incompetence. The desired states are the first two, these are the states of conscious incompetence and conscious competence. Whereas it is not a sin to admit to one's incompetence, it is dangerous not to be aware of one's incompetence. The clear message therefore is to reflect on all your experiences no matter how trivial you may think these experiences are and let self-awareness give direction to your future behaviour. Other ways of enhancing reflective learning are through the concepts of Experiential Learning and Self and Peer Review.

The concept of experiential learning

For a definition of learning, I refer to Kolb (1984), who says that learning is a process whereby knowledge is created through the transformation of experience. This would seem to fit in with Piaget and Inhelder's (1969) concept of schema and adaptation which are discussed in Section I, Chapter 4, where the focus is on thoughts and their reconstruction in an attempt to gain new knowledge. Behaviourists like Watson and Rayner (1920) and Skinner (1974), discussed in Section I, Chapter 8, argue that learning is determined by the way the individual responds to a given stimulus in the environment. One's future behaviour is thus shaped according to the principles of both classical and operant learning. Bandura (1974) argues that some learning take place as a result of watching what others do. The individual basically behaves as the role models have, like in imitating aggressive behaviour. There is without doubt an element of truth in all of those schools of thought. Certainly from Kolb's definition, experience could find its place in all these different theories. Experience in fact is the key issue in the concept of experiential learning. Kolb (1984, p.38) adds that experiential learning emphasises the process of adaptation and learning as opposed to content or outcomes. 'Knowledge is a transformation process, being continually created and recreated not as an independent entity to be acquired or transmitted. . . Learning transforms experience in both its objective and subjective forms.' Henry's (1989) work revealed that for some people all learning, whatever these may be, are experiential. Others remarked that experiential learning is a sequence of stages which includes both experience and reflection.

The types of activity which are considered as experiential learning include:

1   Independent learning, the nature of which is setting up learning contract and students opt to study of their choice, and which has some interest to them.
2   Personal development, this would include anything from group discussion to drama, the main sentiment however is anything which enhances the students' growth and development.
3   Prior learning, the students reflect and evaluate learning which took place previously.
4   Work and community placement, these include the actual hands-on experience.
5   Learning by doing, this involves anything from project work to practical experience.

The foundation of experiential learning is in the work of Lewin (1951), Dewey (1938), and Piaget (1952). Dewey and Lewin shared similar ideas about the concept of experiential learning. I will therefore briefly discuss Lewin's model. As far as Piaget is concerned, Chapter 4 offers an insight into his concept of cognitive development. Lewin's model presents a four-stage learning process, the starting point of which is the concrete experience of the 'here and now kind'. This experience is then analysed and any information which is deduced is used to direct or modify the behaviour of the 'experiencer' (see Figure iv).

Kolb (1984, p.21) states, 'Immediate personal experience is the focal point for learning, giving life, texture, and subjective personal meaning to abstract concepts and at the same time providing a concrete, publicly shared reference point for testing the implications and validity of ideas created during the learning process.' This information is then used to direct one's future course of action.

Concrete experience

Experience is the very foundation of the experiential learning concept. Steinaker and Bell (1979) describe this as the exposure stage, where the student becomes consciously aware of the experience. Experience can be taken to mean any event or activity ranging from structured exercises to, say, watching a video recording. Basically anything which actively involves the student, can be interpreted as an experience. Steinaker and Bell (1979, p.22) state, 'every true teacher realises that in most learning situations – in every new circumstance or activity that involves growth or change – there is an element of uneasiness for the student. This uneasiness, or fear of the unknown, is a necessary part of all experience because, if there is to be a new experience, the student will be following a course he or she cannot completely control and often understand. Although some degree of anxiety may be unavoidable or even desirable, the art and science of teaching require that attention be devoted to this feeling at the start; otherwise, the student may never move beyond the exposure level.'

Observations and reflections

Observations and reflections focus on capturing the essence of the experience in terms of thoughts, feelings and behaviour, before, during and after that experience. These are then made public and shared with student group. Students could ask themselves the following questions: What was the activity about? What was going through my mind before, during and after the activity? There is also an element of sharing notes with other students and establishing any similarities or differences of the experience. This stage is similar to Steinaker and Bell's participation stage, where the focus is in structuring, reviewing, and discussing the information which have been obtained.

Formation of abstract concepts and generalisation

This stage sees the information which is obtained from reflections and observations being used to formulate some theory. Let us say for example the concrete experience was to have been blindfolded and taken for a walk outside for 10 minutes. The information which may be obtained from this experience could be something like feeling frightened, confused, vulnerable, and the feeling of dependency. The 'new theories' which could be deduced from this particular experience may be something like, 'to be blind is to be at the mercy of others' and 'blindness does not necessarily mean loss of visual senses'. This then would form part of the abstract concept from which one can generalise that all those who are blind may suffer a similar experience (note here that the example offered is only an attempt to clarify the concept of experiential learning and the generalisation is only meant in its most superficial form).

Figure iv
*The experimental learning cycle ©
1984. Adapted by permission of
Prentice-Hall, Inc., Upper Saddle
River, NJ.*

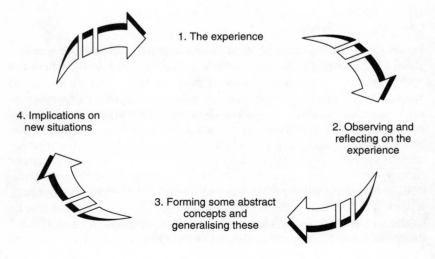

1. The experience

2. Observing and
reflecting on the
experience

3. Forming some abstract
concepts and
generalising these

4. Implications on
new situations

Testing implications of concepts in new situations

New implications for practice can be drawn in that the meaning of blindness can be extended to include lack of information especially when someone is newly admitted to a ward or someone is in a new environment. Equipped with this knowledge, the carer will be better able to offer a good standard of care based on empathic understanding. An element of interaction from the reader is recommended throughout the book because sometimes it is difficult to grasp some sentiments through reading only. Some of these activities need to be processed through the stages of experiential learning.

References

Asch, S.E. (1952). *Social Psychology*. Englewood Cliffs, NJ: Prentice-Hall.

Bandura, A. (1974). Behaviour Theory and the model of man. *American Psychologist*, **29**, 859–869.

Berne, E. (1964). *Games People Play; The Psychology of Human Relationships*. London: Penguin Books.

Buck, R. (1984). *The Communication of Emotion*. New York: Guilford Press.

Brammer, L.M. (1988). *The Helping Relationship; Process and Skills*. London: Allyn and Bacon.

Cartwright, A. (1964). *Human Relations and Hospital Care*. London, UK: Routledge and Kegan Paul.

Condon, W.S. (1980). 'The relation of interactional synchrony to cognitive and emotional process.' In: Key, M.R. (Ed.) *The Relationship of Verbal and Non-Verbal Communication*. The Hague, Paris, New York: Mouton.

Cox, T. (1978). *Stress*. London: MacMillan Education.

Dewey, J, (1938). *Experience and Education*. New York: MacMillan Company.

Egan, G. (1975). *The Skilled Helper*. Monterey, CA: Brooks/Cole.

Erikson, H. (1963). *Childhood and Society*. New York: Norton.

Henry, J. (1989). 'Meaning and practice in experiential learning.' In: Weil, S.W. and McGill, I. (Eds) *Making Sense of Experiential Learning. Diversity in Theory and Practice*. Milton Keynes: The Society for Research into Higher Education and Open University Press.

Hofling, C.K., Brotzman, E., Dalrymple, S., Greaves, N. and Pierce, C.M. (1966). 'An experimental study in nurse–physician relationships.' *Journal of Nervous and Mental Disease*, **143**, 171–180.

Holmes, T. H. and Rahe, R. H. (1967). 'The social readjustment rating scale.' *Journal of Psychosomatic Research*, **11**(2), 213–218.

Kolb, D.A. (1984). *Experiential Learning: Experience as The Source of Learning and Development*. Englewood Cliffs, NJ: Prentice-Hall, Inc.

Kohlberg, L. (1981). *The Philosophy of Moral Development. Essays on Moral Development*, Vol. I. San Francisco, CA: Harper and Row.

Kohler, W. (1925). *The Mentality of Apes*. New York: Harcourt Brace.

Laing, R.D., Phillipson, H. and Lee, A.R. (1966). *Interpersonal Perception. A Theory and Method of Research*. London, UK: Tavistock Publications. New York: Springer Publishing Company.

Lazarus, R.S. and Folkman, S. (1984). *Stress, Appraisal, and Coping*. New York: Springer Publishing Company.

Lewin, K. (1951). *Field Theory in Social Sciences*. New York: Harper and Row.

Luft, J. and Ingham, H. (1955). 'The Johari Window, a graphic model of interpersonal awareness.' In: Luft, J. (1969). *Of Human Interaction*. Palo Alto, CA: National Press.

Maslow, A.H. (1954). *Motivation and Personality*. New York: Harper and Row.

Milgram, S. (1974). *Obedience to Authority: An Experimental View*. London: Tavistock.

Myerscough, P.R. (1992). *Talking with Patients. A Basic Clinical Skill*. Oxford: Oxford University Press.

O'Connor, J. and Seymour, J. (1990). *Introducing Neurolinguistic Programming. Psychological Skills for Understanding and Influencing People*. London: Aquarian.

Pavlov, I.P. (1927). *Conditioned Reflexes*. New York: Oxford University Press.

Piaget, J. (1952). *The Origins of Intelligence in Children*. New York: International Universities Press.

Piaget, J. and Inhelder, B. (1969). *The Psychology of the Child*. London: Routledge and Kegan Paul.

Raphael, W. (1969). *Patients and Their Hospitals*. King Edward's Hospital Funds for London.

Rogers, C.R. (1951). *Client Centred Therapy*. London: Constable.

Seligman, M.E.P. (1975). *Helplessness*. San Francisco, CA: W.H. Freeman.

Selye, H. (1976). *The Stress of Life*, revised edn. New York: McGraw-Hill Book Company.

Skeet, M. (1970). 'Home from Hospital; Dan Mason Nursing Research Committee.' In: Bridge, W. and MacLeod, J.C. (1981). *Communication in Nursing Care*. London: H.M. and M. Publishers.

Skinner, B.F. (1974). *About Behaviourism*. New York: Knopf.

Snyder, M. (1974). 'Self monitoring of expressive behaviour.' *Journal of Personality and Social Psychology*, **30**, 526–537.

Steinaker, N.W. and Bell, M.R. (1979). *The Experiential Taxonomy. A New Approach to Teaching and Learning*. New York: Academic Press.

Stockwell, F. (1984). *The Unpopular Patient*. London: RCN.

Sullivan, H.S. (1953). *The Interpersonal Theory of Psychiatry*. New York: Norton.

Tolman, E.C. (1958). *Essays in Motivation and Learning*. Berkeley: University of California Press.

Watson, J. B. and Rayner, R. (1920). 'Conditioned emotional reactions.' *Journal of Experimental Psychology*, **3**, 1–14.

Watson, J. B. (1930). *Behaviourism*, revised edn. New York: Norton.

Zimbardo, P. (1992). *Psychology of Life*. New York: Harper Collins.

Intrapersonal dynamics and self-awareness

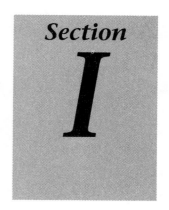

Introduction

It could be argued that the foundation for interpersonal communication rests with intrapersonal dynamics and its interactions with past experiences. Cronen *et al.* (1982) state that the locus of meaning is intrapersonal and the locus of action is interpersonal. The powerhouse of behaviour is undoubtedly within self. From this perspective one could say that what people do and the way they do it are influenced by what goes on inside themselves. One interpretation of what goes on inside oneself' is what is referred to as intrapersonal dynamics, sometimes known as the inner world of the person. One's action becomes clearer as one explores its meaning. In order to understand others, people therefore need to understand themselves in terms of what is going on in the here and now and also what has gone on before. The key to understanding self is clearly from within but always in relation to past experiences. This is simply because self does not exist in a vacuum. Self has always been in constant contact with others, if not physically then psychologically. Laing *et al.* (1966, p.6) stated, 'At the very least, we need concepts which indicate both the interaction and inter-experience of two persons, and help us to understand the relation between each person's own experiences and his own behaviour, always, of course, within the context of the relationship between them.' The starting point of self-knowledge and understanding is with the concept of self-awareness. Condon (1980, p.64) says, 'Much of human life is enslaved to past experiences and this is intertwined with a similar enslavement to culture; both are expressed in the behaviour of our lives. We cannot totally escape them but we can be much more aware of them and their influence.' With this in mind, the voyage begins with an exploration of self-awareness and journeys through to the avenues of effective helping.

A view from within

References

Condon, W.S. (1980). 'The relation of interactional synchrony to cognitive and emotional process.' In: Key, M.R. (Ed.) *The Relationship of Verbal and Non-Verbal Communication*. The Hague, Paris, New York: Mouton.

Cronen, U.E., Pearce, W.B. and Harris, L. (1982). 'The coordinated management of meaning: a theory of communication.' In: Dance, F.E.X. (Ed.) *Human Communication Theory.* New York: Harper & Row.

Laing, R.D., Phillipson, H. and Lee, A.R. (1966). *Interpersonal Perception. A Theory and Method of Research.* London: Tavistock Publications. New York: Springer Publishing Company.

Self-awareness 1

Objectives

After reading this chapter you should be able to:

1   Define self-awareness
2   List some of its major components
3   Explain the dynamic relationships between these components especially within your self
4   Identify the three layers of self-awareness
5   Recognise self-awareness as a prerequisite to health care delivery
6   Realise that self-awareness is a life-long process with limitless boundaries
7   Understand the key role self-awareness plays in interpersonal relationships
8   Discuss how one can become self aware
9   Understand the dynamics between internal response and external behaviour
10   Identify some of these internal responses

In its simplest form self-awareness can be defined as knowing of oneself. This includes amongst many other factors, recognising, acknowledging and challenging as many of our intrapersonal components as we can. Yontef and Simkin (1989) define self-awareness as 'being in touch with one's own existence... Full awareness is the process of being in vigilant contact with the most important events in the individual/environment field with full sensorimotor, emotive, cognitive and energetic support' in

Knowing me knowing you

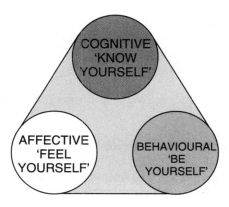

Figure 1.1
The tri-dimensional Cognitive, Affective and Behavioural Components of Self-Awareness

Corsini and Wedding, 1989, p.333). From this perspective, it becomes clear that self-awareness has at least three major components and these are Cognitive, Affective and Behavioural (see Figure 1.1).

Cognitive is taken to mean the thinking aspect, affective is the feeling aspect and behavioural is basically the action one takes. Although these elements are identified separately, this does not mean that each exists in isolation. In fact it could be said that each one exerts its influence on the other two (see Figure 1.2).

Figure 1.2

Interactions between Cognitive, Affective, and Behavioural Components of Self-Awareness

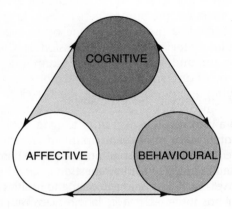

- What I do will influence my thoughts and feelings
- What I think will influence my feelings and behaviour
- What I feel will influence my thoughts and behaviour

Self-awareness therefore, is about recognising, acknowledging, accepting or challenging who we are, what we feel and what we can or cannot do. The word 'challenging' is used tentatively here and as the discussion progresses its meaning will be clarified. Meanwhile have a go at Exercise 1.

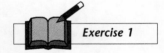 *Exercise 1*

Reflect on your thoughts, feeling and actions and identify one example in each of the following situations

1   Your behaviour has influenced your thoughts
2   Your thought has influenced your behaviour
3   Your behaviour has influenced your feeling
4   Your feeling has influenced your behaviour
5   Your feeling has influenced your thought
6   Your thought has influenced your feeling

Discuss these with a friend, colleague, partner or in a group.

Self-awareness is a personal choice

To discover what one truly is, the feelings one truly feels and the behaviour one truly exhibits, is perhaps a never ending process. However the more knowledge one has of and about oneself the better able one will be at relating to others. To be self-aware or not to be self-aware is a choice one has to make and as Maslow (1968, p.66) said, 'Often it is better not to know, because if you did know, then you would have to stick your neck out.' This can be interpreted to mean that once you are self-aware you cannot ignore what you find, you may have to do something about it. Say for example I become aware of the fact that I have bad breath, it is unlikely that I will carry on as normal. What I will do is to try and take every measure possible to ensure that my bad breath disappears. Within any health care profession, the phrase 'better not to know' is redundant because self-awareness is a prerequisite. One could even say that self-awareness is mandatory for health care professionals. Carers have to be aware of who they are and what they can or cannot do and only then can they hope to be of any value to the clients or patients. Self-awareness is not something that one is born with, one needs to learn not only how to become self-aware but also to be prepared to act on what one finds. Some believe that it is not necessary to read books, attend workshops, or employ an Eastern spiritual discipline in order to increase one's self-awareness because each person has more understanding of him or herself than is being used. The burning question is 'are they aware of the fact that they have more understanding of themselves than is being used?' The answer has to be a categorical 'no' because personal experience suggests that there are many with an attitude of 'I know all there is to know about self-awareness and you can't teach me anything that I don't already know about myself'. Others would comment that it is really common sense anyway. Still some others would say, 'when it comes to talking about myself, I hate it'. For those who believe that they know all there is to know about self-awareness, to them one could say that one can never be overqualified in the field of self-awareness because by its very nature self-awareness has no saturation point. It is in fact a lifelong process which dictates how people grow and develop. The message is clear, if you dare to care, take up the challenge and let self-awareness be the foundation to your existence, learn it and live it, because health care educators cannot gamble on the presumption that you know more about yourself than you let on.

Self-awareness, a prerequisite to caring

Self-awareness, a lifelong process

At the core of the interplay between intra- and interpersonal relationship lies self-awareness. The three different layers in Figure 1.3 represent the depth of one's awareness.

- Layer 1: our more superficial awareness, for example I am aware of my gender, my role etc.

Try and identify some of those things you are superficially aware of.

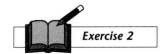

Exercise 2

- Layer 2: our selective awareness. These include the things which I may feel the need to be aware of, for example I need to be aware of my appearance when I go for a job interview. I need to be aware of my relationship with my boss. I need to be aware of my attitude toward a particular subject.

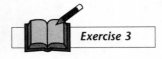

Exercise 3

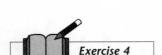

Exercise 4

Identify some of the things you may feel the need to be self-aware of and explore its context.

- Layer 3: our deeper awareness. These are some of the awareness which are only known to myself and to nobody else. For example I am aware of some of my true feelings in relation to a person with an attractive personality. I am also aware of how I feel when I succeed or when the path to the fulfilment of my goal is blocked.

Identify some of your deeper awareness.

Although it is clear that total or complete awareness is an unattainable goal, the more self-aware we are, the better we will be at relating to others. Similarly any sense of self-awareness is better than no self-awareness at all.

Figure 1.3
Self-awareness as the central core of intra- and interpersonal relationships. The three layers are Superficial, Selective and Deeper awareness

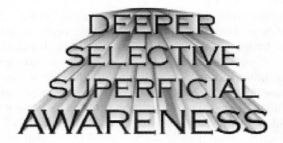

Becoming self-aware

In order to become self-aware, we would need to be able to stand outside of ourselves, reflect on ourselves and evaluate both our intra- and interpersonal elements (see Figure 1.4). Although Figure 1.4 portrays this concept in a rather simplistic way, the actual phenomenon is a rather complex activity. This however does not mean that it is impossible, far from it. In fact, exploration and analysis of our different components can help in achieving this goal. Eric Berne's (1964) model of communication which is

Figure 1.4
Self as an observer and evaluator

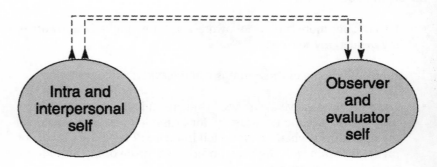

discussed in Chapter 3, shows one possible way through which we can better understand ourselves when we interact with others.

One of the pitfalls of being the observer and evaluator of self is subjectivity. One cannot ignore the fact that one's own subjectivity may dilute one's awareness. For example to further enhance my self-awareness, I need to allow my peers and significant others to occupy the role of observer and evaluator. Here there has to be an element of having to trust the observer to give objective feedback.

Self-awareness can also be promoted by making regular entries in one's journal or diary regarding those critical incidents that one experiences. Critical incidents are taken to mean all those events which make a significant impression in structuring or redirecting one's life map.

The dynamics between internal response and external behaviour

O'Connor and Seymour (1990) focus on internal response and external behaviour as the two distinct parts of self in any interactional process. It could be argued that an awareness of the internal dynamics can enhance the understanding of internal response. If for example I become aware of what is going on in my internal world, I would be in a stronger position to control my external behaviour. This concept will become clearer as the discussion progresses. At this stage however, let us explore some of the elements which form part of this internal dynamic. Exercise 5 is a gradual introduction to the exploration of our inner world.

Part 1: reflect on what goes on within yourself and list as many factors as possible.
Part 2: find a partner, colleague, friend or a group, share some of your thoughts and ideas.

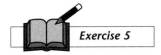

Exercise 5

It could be said that for every interpersonal relationship we have, there is an intrapersonal influence. Expanding on O'Connor and Seymour's (1990) concept of internal response and external behaviour, one could argue that although there is clear evidence of a dynamic relationship between

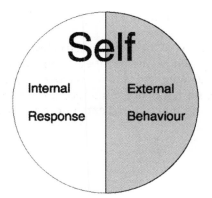

Figure 1.5
After O'Connor and Seymour (1990): Self as consisting of internal response and external behaviour

Figure 1.6
Dynamic interaction between External Behaviour and Internal Response

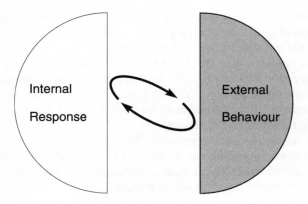

thoughts, feeling and behaviour, nevertheless this does not necessarily mean that one will always behave how one really feels, or for that matter how one really thinks. There are many instances where there is a lack of congruence between thoughts, feeling and behaviour. This is more so when there are conflicts within our intrapersonal dynamics (see Figure 1.6).

Our internal response therefore depends on whether we are able to resolve our internal conflicts. It can be hypothesised that if our internal conflicts are unresolved, then we behave in a manner which is not congruent with either our thoughts or our feelings or both. Penland and Fine (1974) say that it is very difficult for people to change their preconceptions and attitudes, and give up their long-held beliefs. These are instances where there may be a mismatch between thoughts, feelings and behaviour. It would of course be wrong to believe that this incongruency only exists in others. In fact at some time or other, every single individual would have experienced situations where he or she did not behave the way he or she felt or thought.

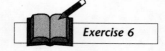

Exercise 6

Reflect on your behaviour and identify one situation when there was incongruency between your:

- Thoughts and behaviour
- Feeling and behaviour
- Feeling and thoughts

Discuss these in pairs or small groups.

A critical look at some of the factors listed below holds the key to understanding why people behave the way they do and also why these elements are considered as the foundations to one's external behaviour. Behaviour is taken to include all forms of communication. Awareness of these elements can reduce both internal and external conflicts. Some of these elements include:

- Thoughts
- Feelings
- Values

- Beliefs
- Attitudes
- Prejudices
- Inner conflicts
- Likes and dislikes
- Opinions and ideas
- Perceptions and inferences
- Preferences for and aversion to
- Past experiences and memories
- Assumptions and interpretations
- Our ability to differentiate and discriminate
- Our sensitivity or resistance to stimuli
- Our fears
- Morals
- Doubts

Some of these factors are discussed in later chapters, meanwhile let us explore the origin of the concept of conscious awareness in Chapter 2.

References

Berne, E. (1964). *Games People Play; The Psychology of Human Relationships*. London: Penguin Books.

Corsini, R.J. and Wedding, D. (1989). *Current Psychotherapies*. Itasca, IU: F.E. Peacock Publishers, Inc.

Cronen, V.E., Pearce, W.B. and Harris, L. (1982). 'The cordinated management of meaning: A theory of communication.' In: Dance F.E.X. (Ed.) (1982). *Toward a Theory of Human Communication*. New York: Holt, Rinehart and Winston.

Maslow, A.H. (1968). *Towards a Psychology of Being*. New York: Van Nostrand.

O'Connor, J. and Seymour, J. (1990). *Introducing Neurolinguistic Programming. Psychological Skills for Understanding and Influencing People*. London: Aquarian.

Penland, P.R. and Fine, S.F. (1974). *Group Dynamics and Individual Development*. New York: Marcel Dekker, Inc.

Yontef, G.M. and Simkin, J.S. (1989). 'Gestalt therapy.' In: Corsini, R.J. and Wedding, D. (Eds) *Current Psychotherapies*. Itasca, IU: F.E. Peacock Publishers, Inc.

Psychoanalytical theory of personality development

2

Objectives

After reading this chapter you should be able to:

1 Identify Freud's notion of levels of awareness
2 Highlight and explain the structure of personality
3 Understand realistic anxiety and neurotic anxiety
4 Define mental defence mechanism, highlight and explain some of these mechanisms and ways of behaving
5 Explain instinct in relation to behaviour and in particular its source, aim, object and impetus
6 Describe the notion of erogenous zones and the stages of psychosexual development
7 Discuss some of the implications of Freud's theory on health care delivery
8 Understand human interaction from Luft and Ingham's (1969) perspective

Sigmund Freud (1856–1939) and the concept of awareness

Level of awareness

The origin of self-awareness can be traced back to Sigmund Freud, who believed that the key to understanding human behaviour rests within the unconscious state of the mind. The starting point of the exploration of the issues of skills, knowledge and awareness therefore is in Freud's psychoanalytical theory, as it came to be known. Psychoanalytical theory was a radical approach to the study of human behaviour in that its focus was on what goes on inside (from a psychological point of view) the person. Hjelle and Ziegler (1992) state that Freud was the first psychologist to show the mind as a battleground for the warring factions of instinct, reason, and conscience. As a result of the interplay between these factions, that is the constant struggle between the instincts, drives and motives, the theory also became known as psychodynamic. The main focus is on the unconscious state of the mind. There are two other states of the mind and these are Conscious and Pre or Subconscious. The mere mention that the majority of people's behaviour seems to emerge from processes which are unavailable to one's awareness may give the impression that this is a load of rubbish, and in fact Freud must have prejudged his readers when he wrote, 'To most people who have been educated in philosophy the idea of anything psychical which is not also conscious is so inconceivable that it seems to them absurd and refutable simply by logic. I believe that this is only because they have never studied the relevant phenomena of hypnosis and dreams which – quite apart from pathological manifestations – necessitate this view' (Freud, 1984, p.351). The idea that the individual functions at three levels of awareness make sense when one considers Exercise 7.

- Identify at least three things which you are conscious of in 'the here and now'
- Reflect on any day of last week and note some of the things you recall from that particular day
- Note one or two things that you did not know about yourself but found out from someone else (that someone, could be an intimate partner or a close friend)

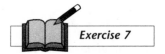

Exercise 7

The three things that I am conscious of at the here and now are:

I am typing these words using only the index finger of each hand.
It is nearly lunch time.
The room that I am in is well lit.

State of conscious awareness

    The things that you have identified would have been similar and this is what Freud called the state of conscious awareness. This means that both you and I are in touch with what is going on at this particular time.

    What I can recall on Tuesday of last week is that I received a copy of Celine Dion's latest compact disc from a very dear friend of mine. I remember asking my youngest son to open the package and we both listened to the first three tracks. Freud believed that this kind of recollection has its origin in the preconscious or subconscious (preconscious and subconscious are basically the same thing). This means that the information is easily retrieved and brought to consciousness whenever one needs to.

State of pre/subconscious awareness

    There are many things I do not know about myself but sometimes my wife or my children point them out to me, for example I am now aware that I have a habit of using a lot of hand movements when I talk. This kind of information unknown to me but through feedback from another person, I am now aware of. Freud argued that such information would have been stored in the unconscious part of people's mind and would be the main determinator of some of the things they say or do. I am sure there are things which we have done during an earlier stage in our lives which are totally lost and irretrievable to our memory. What I mean is, we could have completely forgotten an experience which we had encountered, especially if that experience is too traumatic to remember. It could be argued that this experience is not totally lost, it may well be that it is somewhere in what Freud called the unconscious. Another way of looking at this is that just because you cannot find a particular file in your computer, it does not mean to say that the file does not exist. This idea of unconscious is not as absurd as one may think. It was not so long ago, I received a phone call from someone I used to go to school with when I was a young lad. Up to that time I had completely forgotten her very existence and certainly I cannot even remember what she looked like, but she told

State of unconscious awareness

me she is still as beautiful as ever, come to think of it . . . say no more. In the context of Freud's argument, I am therefore unconscious of certain things that I have lived through.

Three structures of personality

Freud believed that personality has three structures or agencies, Id, Ego, and Super ego and these agencies interact with each other to dictate how an individual behaves. Id is Latin for 'it' and is described as the primitive part of people's personality. Id is also the foundation from which the other two structures, ego and super ego, are developed. Id is believed to be present at birth and is driven solely by biological impulses. Its main purpose in life is to seek pleasure and avoid pain regardless of what the outcome may be. Id functions by the pleasure principle which is the immediate reduction of tension and is wholly instinctive and unconscious. Freud believed that there are two ways the id rids itself of tension and these are reflex action and primary process.

Id, 'The pleasure seeker'

Reflex action

Reflex action is an automatic response which an individual adopts, for example we cough to ease an irritation in our throats, we sneeze to rid ourselves of foreign particles in our noses and tears flow out of our eyes when we have a speck of dirt in them. Similarly when babies' bladders or bowels are full, they have no hesitation in emptying them wherever they happen to be.

Primary process

Primary process is a much more controlled mechanism. Let us say the babies are hungry. Reflex action is not useful because it cannot bring food to them to satisfy their hunger, instead the id will conjure up a mental picture of something which will satisfy the babies' hunger, for example their milk bottles or mothers' breasts. The potential problem of the primary process is that these babies could end up in a fantasy world if they always use mental imagery to relieve internal tension. One of the tasks which faces these babies therefore is to learn to delay gratification of the primary needs. As they grow older they soon realise that their biological impulses cannot be satisfied as and when they want, for example if they have the impulse to empty their bladders or bowels, they cannot just micturate or excrete wherever they are, they have to wait for the appropriate place. This is where the second agency of the mind, the ego, comes into play.

Ego 'The rational thinker'

The Ego which is Latin for 'I', helps the individual to suppress these impulses until the appropriate time or place in which to release them. Ego functions on reality principle and is very much a conscious experience. Ego is the rational part of one's personality. Its main responsibility is to seek ways that the desires of the id can be expressed without interfering with societal boundary. The ego functions by recognising the difference between what exists in the mind and in the outside world. Whereas the id functions through a primary thinking process, the ego adopts a secondary process and this is based on rational thinking.

Super ego 'The perfection seeker'

The Super ego is the last structure to develop and as the child grows older he or she is still influenced by significant others and learns what is right and what is wrong. The super ego is said to function on the moral principle and is seen as the complete opposite to the id. It aims to seek perfection and ideals. It is said to be puritanical in nature. The exerting influence of the super ego is such that it wants the ego to seek perfection rather than function according to the demands of reality. The super ego is divided into two subsections and these are conscience and ego ideal.

Conscience is developed though parental control, mainly through punishment. For example if the child misbehaves then he or she is punished. *Conscience*

Ego ideal is opposite to the conscience in that it is concerned with reward. Here there is parental approval for good behaviour. *Ego ideal*

The id is described as the foundation upon which both the ego and super ego rest. The ego is mostly conscious, a greater portion of the super ego rests in the unconscious, whereas the whole of the id resides in the unconscious. Freud in fact argued that people's level of conscious awareness is only 20 per cent compared to their whole behaviour. This suggests that we may not be aware of most of the things that we say or do. Our level of consciousness has been likened to an iceberg, what we see above water is that portion of our consciousness and the massive portion which is submerged is the unconscious.

Anxiety and realistic anxiety

According to Hjelle and Ziegler (1992) Freud's conception of anxiety is that it is a function of the ego to alert the person of the impending danger which must be avoided. Anxiety therefore can be seen as a person's way of reacting to a threatening situation in what could be called a socially acceptable manner. Freud used the term realistic anxiety to suggest the reaction which anyone would portray in the presence of a threatening or fearful situation like having to sit an examination or taking the driving test. 'Realistic anxiety strikes us as something very rational and intelligible. We may say of it that it is a reaction to the perception of an external danger – that is an injury which is expected or foreseen. It is connected with the flight reflex and it may be regarded as a manifestation of the self-preservative instinct' (Freud, 1973, p.441). The origin of anxiety is as Freud saw it, in the 'act of birth' which brings about unpleasurable feelings. Hjelle and Ziegler's (1992, pp.102–103) note 'the experience of biological separation from the mother acquires a traumatic quality so that later separations . . . produce strong anxiety reactions'.

A second type of anxiety which Freud identified is neurotic anxiety, *Neurotic anxiety* where the desire to express some of the impulses of the id may become conscious. Here there is an element of being afraid of what may happen if the id is allowed to have free expression. The consequence may be too frightening to even think of. Having said that some of these behaviours can be seen as causing no serious harm or disruption like those streakers at sports venues. Generally the ego prevents such behaviour from happening by adopting certain strategies to deal with this potential danger. The ego is also faced with the possible threat of punishment from the super *Moral anxiety* ego whenever the id seeks active expression of immoral thoughts or acts. It is as though the ego faces a dilemma, and the term moral anxiety applies. According to Freud there are certain defences which need to be set up in order to deal with these anxieties and these are commonly known as mental defence mechanisms.

Anxiety and defence mechanisms

Mental defence mechanism is defined as a psychological strategy which is employed by the ego to protect the person from anxiety or internal conflict. Numerous mechanisms have been identified and although most of them are employed unconsciously, there are some which are used consciously, suppression being one of them. Mental defence mechanisms include the following.

Denial

Denial is a way of avoiding or escaping from certain unpleasant realities of life by behaving as if they have not occurred or are not happening. This is frequently displayed when, for example, someone has failed an exam. A typical reaction to this bad news may be, 'I am sure they have got my name mixed up. Surely it can't be me.' This is a typical defence which is adopted as a reaction to a loss and is seen as the first stage of the grieving process by Khubler-Ross (1969).

Displacement

Displacement can be described as the transfer of emotions associated with a particular object (person or situation) onto another non-threatening object. An example would be, 'my boss tells me off for not doing my job properly, I can't express my true feelings there and then, so I go home and shout or scream at my family'.

Projection

Projection is described as the unconscious rejection of emotional manifestation within oneself and attributing the same emotional manifestation to another person. For example 'I don't like you and I put the blame on you and accuse you of not liking me'.

Introjection

Introjection is described as the taking on of the values or personal attributes of significant others and behaving as if these are really one's own. For example 'my mother values education and believes that everything else comes second. My values may be completely opposite to hers nevertheless because of my emotional tie with her and what's more important I wouldn't like to be on the wrong side of her. I take on her strong values and behave as if these were mine.'

Suppression

Suppression is described as the act of consciously putting something (this could be a trauma, bad memories or a negative experience) out of one's awareness. An example would be refusing to think about your poor financial situation at your birthday party or when you are on holiday.

Reflect and recall any defence mechanisms you may have used in the past and discuss these with your colleagues or in a group.

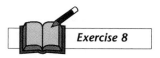

Exercise 8

Instinct and behaviour

Freud argued that the reason people behave the way they do is because of their instincts, drives and motives. The implication is that it is these instincts and drives which motivate people's behaviour. Behaviour therefore is contingent on motives. Instincts are unlearned patterns of behaviour, for example 'I don't learn to be hungry, nor do I learn to empty my bowels, I just know how and what it feels to be hungry or when my bladder is full'. There are two principal types of instincts and these are life instinct and death instinct.

Eros

Life instinct is also referred to as Eros, and is associated with all those behaviours which seek to maintain life and sexual gratification through the expression of sexual energy. The energy force behind the sexual instinct is known as libido.

Thanatos

Death instinct is known as Thanatos, and is associated with all those behaviours which seek to terminate life. The death instinct shows itself through such behaviours as aggression, depression, suicide and homicide. In contrast to life instinct, where the goal of life is to survive and procreate, the goal of death instinct is death and destruction. The implication is that in one way or another, we all have an unconscious wish to die. According to Hjelle and Ziegler (1992), the concept of instinct have four features. These are source, aim, object and impetus.

    The source of the life instincts rests in neurophysiology and that of the death instincts is not quite clear.   *Source*

    The aim of any instinct is to destroy itself. If for example my instinct is hunger, the aim of my hunger is to reduce or appease it.   *Aim*

    Object is the thing which will actually provide the satisfaction of my instinct, in this case food.   *Object*

    Impetus can be seen as the lengths to which a person will go to satisfy his or her instinct. It is basically the strength of the force it will take to gratify the instinct.   *Impetus*

Main sex instincts

Freud argued that there are more than one sex instinct, these are in fact spread over different regions of the body and are called erogenous zones. These include the ears, eyes, and breasts. The mains ones however, are:

- oral, which is the mouth
- anal, which is the anus
- genitals, which are the genital organs

Erogenous zones

Freud's argument is that these erogenous zones are potential sources of tension, which can only be relieved through manipulation of these areas. For example eating, biting and sucking will provide relief and pleasure of the oral zone, defecating provides anal pleasure, and masturbating provides genital relief and pleasure. Sexual pleasure through the erogenous zones serves as a foundation for Freud's concept of personality development. Freud stated that personality development follows a series of stages and most of these stages are linked with sexual gratification, hence the term Psychosexual Stages. The resolution or fixation of these stages (this means their successful or unsuccessful completion), leads to the establishment of certain personality traits and characteristics. The concepts of Frustration and Overindulgence are significant to the outcomes of these stages. Frustration suggests that the psychosexual needs are hindered, whereas overindulgence indicates an element of lack of control over these stages. The individual is basically free to engage in the activities for as long as he or she wants. Other concepts which are relevant to the psychosexual stages are Fixation and Regression. Fixation means that development stops at a particular point along the stages. For example the individual may not be able to go any further than the anal stage. Regression on the other hand means going back to an early psychosexual stage, for example faced with a conflict situation the individual may revert back to the oral stage, where he or she may suck his or her thumb or bite his or her nails. A classic example of regression is when a child starts to wet the bed after having had full bladder control, but the behaviour is as a response to say, the birth of a younger brother or sister. The child fears that he will not have the love of his parents. These psychosexual stages are identified as oral, anal, phallic, latency and genital.

Psychosexual stages

Frustration and overindulgence

Fixation and regression

Oral stage

The oral stage is from birth to approximately 18 months. The erogenous zones are focused around the mouth and on the lips. Gratification is obtained from eating, sucking, biting and other such like behaviour. Freud stated, 'if an infant could speak, he would no doubt pronounce the act of sucking at his mother's breast by far the most important in his life. . . Sucking at his mother's breast is the starting point of the whole of sexual life' (Freud, 1973, p.356). The oral stage is believed to be an important erogenous zone throughout life, and this includes adult life. According to Freud, if infants are given either excessive or insufficient amounts of stimulation they are likely to become an oral-passive personality type when they grow into adulthood. This personality type is characterised by being cheerful and optimistic. These people expect everyone to pamper them, and are always wanting approval for what they do. Psychologically these individuals are gullible, passive, immature and extremely dependent. The oral stage is marked by a second phase which begins when the infant starts teething. This is referred to as oral-aggressive or oral-sadistic and is characterised by biting and chewing as a means of expressing frustration caused by delayed gratification. Argumentative, pessimistic, sarcastic, and cynical are amongst the traits of adult behaviour which suggest 'fixation'.

Anal stage

The anal stage is 18 months to approximately 3 years. According to Freud, the anus becomes the focus of the erogenous zone. The child is believed to derive pleasure from both retention and expulsion of faeces. 'I know you have been wanting for a long time to interrupt me and exclaim: "Enough of these atrocities! You tell us that defecating is a source of sexual satisfaction, and already exploited in infancy! That faeces is a valuable substance and that the anus is a kind of genital!" . .No, Gentlemen. . . Why should you not be aware that for a large number of adults, homosexual and heterosexual alike, the anus does really take over the role of the vagina in sexual intercourse?' (Freud, 1973, pp.357–358). The suggestion is that if the child is brought up in an environment where toilet training is rigid and too controlled, the child stands to develop an anal retentive personality type, which is characterised by being obstinate, orderly, punctual and stingy. Another type of anal personality develops as a result of strict control over toilet training and this is anal-expulsive. This is expressed through such behaviours as destructiveness, disorderliness, impulsivity, and cruelty. According to Hjelle and Ziegler (1992) such an individual tends to see others primarily as objects to be possessed.

Anal retentive and anal expulsive

Phallic stage

The phallic stage is 3 years to 6 years. Here the erogenous zone has moved to the genitals and stimulation of these leads to sexual pleasure. A very important development occurs during this stage, Freud called this the Oedipus complex. Freud in fact said that what he had in mind is rivalry in love with a clear emphasis on the child's sex. The small boy will have already started to develop a special kind of affection for his mother, whom he sees as belonging to him. He sees his father as a rival who has a claim for his sole possession. Similarly the little girl sees her mother as the rival for her father's affection. The name Oedipus is derived from Sophocles' fictitious play, where King Oedipus Rex, unknowingly murdered his father and had sex with his mother. This type of conflict in girls is referred to as the Electra complex, a term which was used by Jung. Electra is a Greek character who persuaded her brother to kill their mother and her lover to avenge their father's death. The resolution of the Oedipus complex is said

Oedipus and Electra complex

Resolution of Oedipus complex

Castration anxiety

Resolution of Electra complex

Penis envy

to take place when the boy is about 5 to 7 years old. The basic conflict is getting rid of father and being with mother, however when the little boy realises that he does not stand a chance against his father, he develops a fear that his father may punish him for the way he feels towards his mother. The child in fact fears that his father may cut off his penis, this therefore leads to what Freud called castration anxiety. The boy deals with this by repressing this love for his mother and forgetting about it. He starts to identify with his father and Hjelle and Ziegler (1992) explain that this identification with the aggressor serves several functions which include, being an avenue for the boy to experience what it feels like to be a male and how he needs to behave and sharing the mother's love.

Resolution of the Electra complex is different to that of the Oedipus complex. Here as soon as the little girl discovers that she is different to little boys, in that she does not have a penis, she becomes hostile towards her mother and blames her for taking away her penis in retribution for some bad things which she may have done. Freud said that the little girl suffers from what is called 'penis envy'. One of the versions of how the girl overcomes the Electra complex can be deduced from Freud's quote, 'In my experience it seldom goes beyond the taking of her mother's place and the adopting of a feminine attitude towards her father. Renunciation of the penis is not tolerated by the girl without some attempt at compensation. She slips – along the line of a symbolic equation, one might say – from the penis to a baby' (Freud, 1972, p.321). The implication is that she wants to have a baby from her father but gradually gives up this idea because she realises that this will never be. But still these two wishes which are, to possess a penis and to have a baby, remain in the unconscious and these actually help to prepare the woman for her later sexual role.

According to Hjelle and Ziegler (1992) fixation at the phallic stage leads the male to behave in a brash and boastful manner. Phallic types try hard to be successful and success represents having the upper hand over the opposite-sexed-parent. Phallic fixation in women is characterised by being flirtatious, seductive, and promiscuous.

Latency

The latency stage is 6/7 years to 11/12 years. This is the only stage which shows a temporary freeze from sexual gratification and no involvement of any erogenous zones. Pleasure is obtained through sports and any related activities, and being with peers.

Genital stage

The genital stage (puberty onward) is described as the stage which suggests complete satisfaction of the sexual instinct. The person is ready in every aspect to engage in sexual intercourse. Initially the young person focuses his or her interest towards members of the same sex, then gradually shifts to members of the opposite sex.

The implications for health care delivery

If what Freud said is true, that is, people are only aware of roughly 20 per cent of what they say or do, then it does not bear thinking of the potential damage that could be caused when health carers interact with clients or patients. For example I may not be aware of my true likes and dislikes when I am actually in the helper role. I may believe that I am doing it right, when I may in fact be quite wrong. Similarly I could be employing one or more of those mental defence mechanisms during an interaction with others and my lack of awareness will make it such that I am basically rendered incompetent (unconscious incompetence). In some ways Freud's concept of the levels of awareness can be linked with the concept of the Johari Window.

Johari Window: a model for self-awareness

Johari Window is included (a concept by Joseph Luft and Harry Ingham) because as Luft (1969) said, it deals with awareness in human behaviour; he identified seven central issues, four of which are highlighted below:

- awareness and consciousness are uniquely human attributes. The sentiment here is that these are extremely important factors in terms of human interaction
- intrapersonal and interpersonal issues are united and lend themselves to be viewed together
- the model can be applied to any human interaction
- it is content free, which suggests that it can be viewed from any perspective of personality development

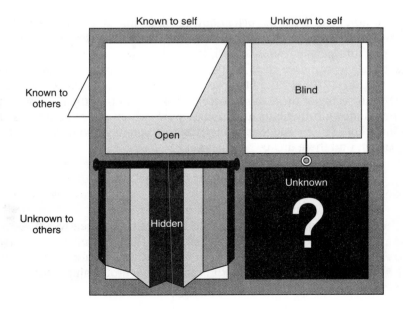

Figure 2.1
The Johari Window which shows the four facets of self

Luft and Ingham (1955) presented their classic model, the Johari Window, where the dynamics of a person's being is seen to consist of four quadrants. 'The four quadrants represent the total person in relation to other persons. The basis for division into quadrants is awareness of behaviour, feelings, and motivation' (Luft, 1969, p.13). Each quadrant is labelled according to the level of the person's awareness (see Figure 2.1).

Quadrant 1 is seen as the Open or visible part of self, behaviour, feeling, and motivation, which is known to both self and others. Try Exercise 9.

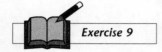

Exercise 9

List some of your behaviour, feelings, thoughts and motivation which are known to both yourself and others.

Quadrant 2 is the part which is Blind to self (behaviour, feelings and motivation which we are unaware of) but others are aware of. Bad breath is probably the most common example one can think of. Other examples include:

- the fact that we may be critical of people and not being aware of it
- our peculiarities, mannerisms
- the fact that we may repeat ourselves without knowing it
- others may see us blush
- the way we walk
- what our voice sounds like

Quadrant 3 is that aspect (behaviour, feelings and motivation) which is hidden to others but known to self. Some examples include strong emotional feeling for others, secrets or hidden messages. Try Exercise 10.

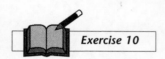

Exercise 10

Identify for yourself some of the behaviour, thoughts, feelings and motivations which are known to you but not to others.

Quadrant 4 is the area (behaviour, feelings and motivation) which is unknown to both self and others. Very often when discussing this particular quadrant people usually ask, 'if this is unknown to both self and others, then how come we know of such an area?' The answer is quite simple really. Luft (1970, p.12) states 'we can assume their existence because eventually some of these things become known, and we then realise that these unknown behaviours and motives were influencing relationships all along'. Luft (1969) suggests some ways of detecting what lies in the unknown and these are:

- confirmation after the fact, where a sudden change of behaviour could be linked to one's predisposition. It is as if it was always there but did not actually surface until now
- alcohol, drugs or even fever could lead a person to behave differently to his or her usual way of behaving
- hypnosis
- different behaviour as a result of irreversible brain injury and this could be compared to premorbid behaviour

- projective techniques such as the Rorschach inkblot test or the Thematic Apperception Test, could reveal the things about oneself which nobody knew, not even oneself
- daydreams as well as night dreams

The explanation of the concept of the Johari Window has been rather simplistic, however this should not detract from the fact that if each and everyone of us were to critically analyse our behaviour and our being, we would most certainly come to the same conclusion as Luft and Ingham (1955). 'Like the happy centipede, many people get along fine working with others without thinking about which foot to put forward' (Luft, 1970, p.11). This is okay as long as things go well, but as soon as things start to get difficult, we would then have wished to know more about the dynamics of person to person interaction and in particular the level of our own awareness. To this end therefore one could say that self-awareness is the fulcrum of both intra- and interpersonal relationships. Self-awareness remains one of the most powerful tools for health care delivery. The Johari Window is explored further in Section III, Chapter 19. The dynamics of interaction are made visible through Berne's (1964) concept of transactional analysis and this is discussed in the chapter to follow.

References

Berne, E. (1964). *Games People Play; The Psychology of Human Relationships.* London: Penguin Books.

Freud, S. (1972). *On Sexuality. Three Essays on the Theory of Sexuality and Other Works.* London: Penguin Books.

Freud, S. (1973). *Introductory Lectures on Psychoanalysis.* London: Penguin Books.

Freud, S. (1984). *On Metapsychology.* London: Penguin Books.

Hjelle, L.A. and Ziegler, D.J. (1992). *Personality Theories. Basic Assumptions, Research, and Applications.* New York: McGraw-Hill International Editions.

Khubler-Ross, E. (1969). *On Death and Dying.* New York: MacMillan.

Luft, J. (1969). *Of Human Interaction.* Palo Alto, CA: National Press.

Luft, J. (1970). *Group Process. An Introduction to Group Dynamics.* Palo Alto, CA: National Press.

Luft, J. and Ingham, H. (1955). 'The Johari Window, A graphic model of interpersonal awareness.' In: Luft, J. (1969). *Of Human Interaction.* Palo Alto, CA: National Press.

Transactional analysis 3

Objectives

After reading this chapter you should be able to:

1 Explain what transactional analysis is and state its components
2 Describe each of these components
3 Define the terms ego state, stroke, hunger, and transaction
4 Explain contamination and exclusion
5 Discuss the notion of games and explain some of the commonest games people play
6 Explain life script and behaviour
7 Understand how a knowledge of the concept of transactional analysis can enhance care delivery

Eric Berne (1910–1970)

Transactional analysis is a theory of personality which was originated in the 1950s by Eric Berne. Transactional analysis, commonly known as TA, is described as a method through which most, if not all, forms of person to person communication can be systematically analysed. TA is also used as a tool for therapeutic intervention. Therapeutic intervention is taken to mean that it helps to enhance clients' growth, development and personal autonomy. Client in this context is taken to mean anyone who is in need of health care, whatever the degree may be. The assumptions which underpin transactional analysis include the following sentiments.

Assumptions of transactional analysis

1 People are okay, this suggests an inherent goodness in people
2 People can solve their problems
3 People can work together
4 People can take responsibility for themselves
5 People know what they need but may need help in expressing these needs

The basic concept of TA can be seen through four components and these are:

Components of TA

1 Structure: analysis of the structure of one's personality
2 Transaction: analysis of what one says or does in relation to others
3 Games: analysis of one's ulterior motives in the way one acts
4 Script: analysis of one's specific life dramas that one engages in

Structural analysis

Structural analysis offers a way of finding out 'Who we are?' and 'Why we behave the way we do?' Here the focus is on analysing one's thoughts, feelings and behaviour. From Berne's (1961) perspective, one's intrapersonal structure is composed of three basic components and collectively they are referred to as ego states. From a practical perspective, an ego state can be described as 'a system of feelings which motivates a related set of behaviour patterns' (Berne, 1961, p.17). In its simplest form, an ego state is a state of mind. The three primary ego states are identified as: Parent, Adult and Child, represented as three circles touching but not overlapping each other (see Figure 3.1).

The implication is that each and every individual has these three ego states and when people interact with each other they do so through these channels. Like a car with its different sets of gears to suit different conditions, people interact with their different set of ego states according to the perception of their needs or according to how they feel. The ego states function independently of one another, with clear boundaries. 'Each ego state has its own observable mannerisms, a special repertoire of words, thoughts, emotions, body postures, gestures, voice tones, and expressions' (Dusay and Dusay, 1989, p.406).

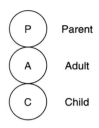

Figure 3.1
The structure of self through the three primary ego states

Parent ego state

The parent ego state reflects the sentiments of one's attitudes, values, beliefs and morals. People acquire these from their parents. It functions in two ways, on the one hand it promotes growth and development and on the other it tends to criticise and seeks to control. It is for this reason that the parent ego state is always diagrammatically represented as one circle divided into two distinct parts, as shown in Figure 3.2. The terms Critical Parent and Nurturing Parent are used to distinguish the two secondary ego states of the parent. Some prefer to substitute critical parent for control parent because the former can portray the parent in a negative way when in fact no one ego state is seen as better than the others. What needs to be said however, is that one ego state may be more appropriate in certain situation than others. According to James and Jongeward (1971), when people are acting, thinking, feeling as they see their parents to be doing, they are in fact in their Parent ego state. Parent ego state parallels Freud's concept of super ego in that there is an element of morality.

Figure 3.2
The two secondary ego states of the parent

Reflect on some of the ways your parent(s) acts, thinks, feels, and check out if any of these are reflected in the way you act, think and feel.

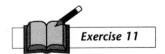

Exercise 11

Adult ego state

The Adult ego state can be likened to a computer in its function of information processing. It is said to deal with rationality and logic reasoning. Unlike the parent ego state the adult ego state has no secondary ego state, hence the rationality of one's behaviour when the adult ego state is in action. In many ways the adult ego state is similar to Freud's concept of the ego because behaviour is mainly based on logic reasoning. Again James and Jongeward's sentiment suggests that when the person deals with current reality, collecting facts and computing objectively, they are in their adult ego state.

Child ego state

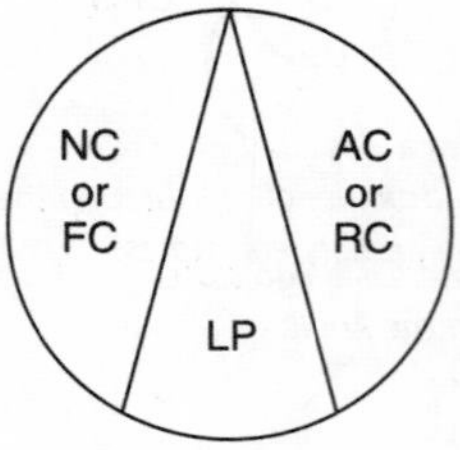

The behaviour of one's Child ego state is said to be similar to that of one's actual child regardless of one's age. It is described as being spontaneous, fun loving, emotional and has a desire to seek pleasure. It is also an individual's most vulnerable part. It can be appealing and attractive and can be regarded as the feeling part of self. The Child ego state consists of three secondary ego states and these are identified as Natural or Free Child, Adapted/Rebellious Child and Little Professor (see Figure 3.3). The Natural Child is seen as the unrestraining and unbounded aspect of one's personality, in many ways similar to Freud's concept of the Id. The Adapted Child on the other hand is an individual's compliant and co-operative side. There is an element here of doing what significant others want the person to do and in a way the individual tries to fit into the needs of the family and society. Sometimes however, parental influences and demands can be too much for the Adapted Child to accept. When this happens, the person switches to the Rebellious Child ego state, and this is demonstrated through non-compliance. The Little Professor is described as a person's intuitive self. One may for example feel that something is true, but has no way of proving it. Berne (1961, p.207) said 'this kind of shrewdness in appraising and manipulating personal relationships is an important aspect of the growing child's personality, . . . since it requires sensitive and objective data processing based on experience. . . It often has a disconcerting and sometimes withering accuracy, as shown in many anecdotes about children.' One way of checking out our child ego state is to reflect on the way we behaved when we were children.

The very nature of human behaviour suggests that an individual can behave one way in one situation and a different way in other situations. One can plot, from an egogram, the qualitative differences in behaviour based on different situations, for example it is most certain that my behaviour is different at home than it is when I am at work. Whereas at work I may confine myself to my professional boundaries, at home I am free to behave in any way I choose. You will, as a general rule, find that your ego states vary significantly from work to your home situation.

Contamination

Two concepts relevant to ego states need to be introduced here, these are Contamination and Exclusion. Contamination suggests that the Adult ego state is interfered with by either the Parent or the Child or by both the Parent and the Child ego states (see Figure 3.4) and note the overlapping parent's circle onto the adult. When the Parent ego state contaminates the Adult ego state, this means that the latter cannot function without being biased by the former. This dynamic leads the individual to behave in a prejudicial manner.

The contamination of the Adult ego state by the Child means that the former cannot function without being biased by the latter. This dynamic leads the individual to suffer from irrational fears.

Figure 3.3
Child with its three secondary ego states. Free or Natural child. Adapted or Rebellious child and the Little Professor

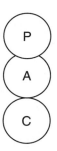

Figure 3.4
The rational Adult ego state is contaminated by the parent

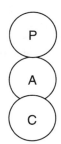

Figure 3.5
Child ego state contaminating the Adult ego state

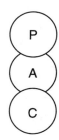

Figure 3.6
Both Parent and Child ego states contaminating the Adult

The contamination of the Adult ego state by both the Parent and the Child means that the person is left in a confused state and may lead the individual to suffer from hallucinations.

Exclusion suggests that an individual does not make full use of all his or her three ego states (see Figures 3.7, 3.8, 3.9).

Exclusion

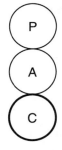

Figure 3.7
An individual functioning by using the Child ego state only

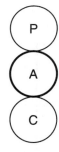

Figure 3.8
An individual functioning by using Adult ego state only

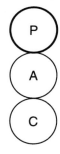

Figure 3.9
An individual functioning by using the Parent ego state

Exclusion can be interpreted in two ways. Firstly, it can be taken to mean that the individual is using only one of his or her ego states, for example using the Child ego state permanently, using the Adult ego state permanently and using the Parent ego state permanently. An understanding of each of the functions of the particular ego states enables one to recognise these individuals during an interaction. According to James and Jongeward (1971), a person who uses only the Parent ego state or the Child ego state and does not use the Adult ego state is likely to be seriously disturbed. This suggests that this particular person is not in touch with what is currently happening, and is not reality testing in the here and now. Similarly a person who does not use both the Parent and Child, but who uses the Adult may be a bore or a robot, without feeling or passion.

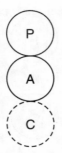

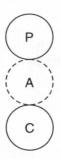

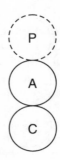

Figure 3.10
The Child ego state is redundant

Figure 3.11
The Adult ego state is redundant

Figure 3.12
The Parent ego state is redundant

Secondly, exclusion can be taken to mean that the person does not use one particular ego state as shown by the dotted circles in Figure 3.10, 3.11 and 3.12.

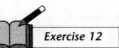 **Exercise 12**

Based on a sum total of behaviour of 100 per cent, plot your individual ego state in both situations, i.e. At home and at work.

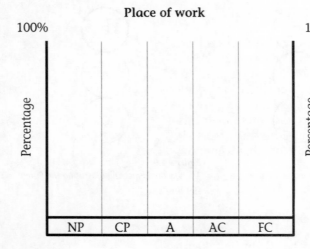

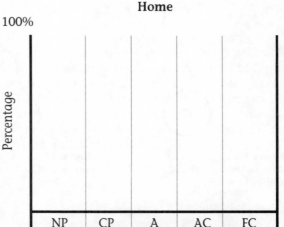

KEY: NP   = Nurturing Parent
        CP   = Critical Parent
        A   = Adult
        AC   = Adaptive Child
        FC   = Free Child

Transactionalysis proper

Berne argued that the need to be recognised and touched has both psychological and biological implications. Each and every individual seeks the satisfaction of being touched and recognised. Being recognised by others suggests that an individual is being acknowledged as existing, this is like giving the 'I know you are there' message. Any such act, be it verbal or non-verbal is described as a stroke. Stroke is defined as one unit of recognition. The need for such strokes are called hungers. Initially, strokes take the form of hungers. James and Jongeward (1971) argued that if an infant is deprived of touch in the early stage of life, his growth and development will be impaired and deterioration will even be to the point of death. 'As a child grows older, the early primary hunger for actual physical touch is modified and becomes recognition hunger. A smile, a nod, a word, a frown, a gesture eventually replace some touch strokes.' James and Jongeward (1971, p.46). It needs to be pointed out at this stage that strokes can be both positive and negative. People who receive positive strokes will develop a healthy emotional state because the message that they pick up is that they are okay. Those who receive negative strokes could grow up to be emotionally unstable, with the message that they are not okay.

'If you touch me soft and gentle
If you look at me and smile
If you listen to me talk sometimes before you talk
I will grow, really grow.'
            Bradley (aged 9 years), James and Jongeward (1971, p.44).

Bradley's sentiment captures the essence of the need for positive stroking. Reflecting on the concept of ego states, one notes that Berne (1961) actually described the structure of personality as having a set of three ego states, Parent, Adult and Child (PAC). This means that when two people are interacting with one another, 'psychologically speaking . . . there are actually six structured ego states present and these ego states may transact and communicate with one another' (Dusay and Dusay, 1989, p.407). They do so in a variety of combinations and these fall into three main categories or types. They are:

* complimentary
* crossed and
* ulterior

Complimentary transactions

Berne (1964) saw the simplest form of transactions as those where the adult ego state of both people interact with one another. I could for example say, hello to you, and in return you say hello to me (see Figure 3.13). This would suggest that my Adult is addressing your Adult and my stroke is acknowledged by your Adult, and in turn your Adult responds to my Adult. This is called a complementary transaction because the response comes from the same ego state which has been addressed. Other permutations of complementary transaction include Parent to Parent, Child to Child, Parent to Child and vice versa. If my Parent ego state was to address

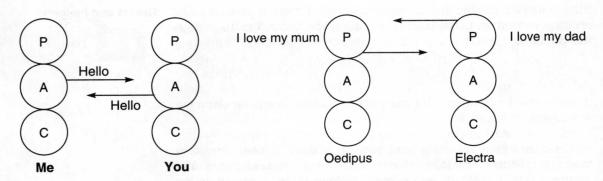

Figure 3.13
A 'You and Me interaction'

Figure 3.14
An exchange between Oedepus and Electra

your Parent ego state and your Parent ego state responds, this would be another complementary transaction. Imagine this hypothetical interaction between two lecturers, let us call them Oedipus and Electra for the fun of it (see Figure 3.14).

Figure 3.15 illustrates an hypothetical interaction between two people, and again for the fun of it let us call them Drink and Drive as an attempt to demonstrate a Child to Child interaction. Similarly let us look at a scenario between a father and a son in Figure 3.16.

Figure 3.15
Drink interacting with Drive

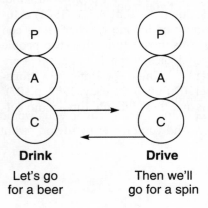

Figure 3.16
A father and son interaction

Find yourself a partner and choose a topic where there is likely to be an element of 'agreeing with each other' and spend about 5 to 10 minutes talking to each other.

Exercise 13

At the end of the time, reflect on what you have been doing in terms of content of speech and exhibited behaviours.

Now try and imagine that if time was not an issue how long could you have gone on talking for.

The truth is that you could have gone on talking for a very long time and in fact Berne (1964) stated that the first rule of communication is that communication will proceed smoothly so long as the transactions are complimentary. In principle therefore communication can last indefinitely. In this situation the topic of the conversation would seem to be irrelevant, as Berne said, people could be doing anything from engaging in critical gossip to playing together.

Find yourself a partner and this time choose a topic where you are most likely to disagree with each other and spend about 5 or 10 minutes talking to each other.

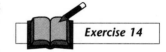

Exercise 14

Once you have finished, again reflect over the last 5 or 10 minutes, whichever time is appropriate and note both your behaviours, let this include your verbal and non-verbal behaviour. It would also be interesting to establish what were the topic or topics of your conversation.

Crossed transactions

Hopefully this exercise would have introduced you to the basic principles of a crossed transaction. A crossed transaction therefore occurs when a message sent from one ego state gets a totally unexpected response, which is usually negative and critical. If for example I was to say to you, 'would you mind giving me a lift in your car?' And you answer by saying, 'what

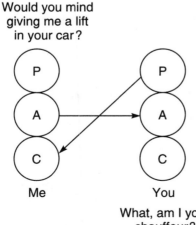

Would you mind
giving me a lift
in your car?

Me   You

What, am I your
chauffeur?

Figure 3.17
*A crossed Adult to Adult and
Parent to Child transaction*

am I, your chauffeur?' This would be seen as a crossed transaction. This scenario is represented in Figure 3.17. In this instance my Adult ego state makes an attempt to stimulate your Adult ego state, your response however comes from your Parent ego state and is directed at my Child ego state. The two arrows cross each other. When this happens, communication is either broken off or the topic of conversation changes. You may have found that out for yourself in Exercise 14.

Again there are numerous permutations to this type of interaction. Figure 3.17 shows Adult to Adult and Parent to Child crossed transaction, in fact according to Stewart and Joines (1987), Berne calculated 72 possible permutations. You will be glad to know that I have no intention of searching for those combinations, having said that perhaps you could take on the challenge and identify them.

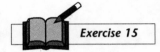

Exercise 15   Identify as many possible combinations of crossed transactions as you can and draw a transactional diagram for each of your transactions.

Ulterior transactions

An ulterior transaction involves more than two ego states at the same time. A typical example of an ulterior transaction can be seen in the following interaction between Paul and Jan.

Paul: Would you like to come and see my etchings?
Jan: I'd like that very much.
Taken at face value this transaction is represented in Figure 3.18.

Figure 3.18
The start of an ulterior transaction

Figure 3.19
Shows the hidden meaning of what Paul and Jan really mean

Paul: Come and let's make love
Jan: Let's

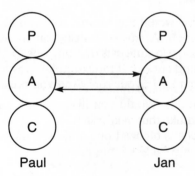

The overt message is being transmitted from adult to adult. Now let us suppose both Paul and Jan had ulterior motives for the stimulus and response transactions. And hypothetically let us say that Paul and Jan's Ulterior Stimulus and Response transactions are sexually orientated and this can be represented in Figure 3.19.

Duplex transaction

This transaction suggests that there are two messages being transmitted at the same time. The first one is overt in that it is what can be heard but it carries a completely different meaning altogether. What is heard therefore is an adult to adult transaction. The hidden or covert messages are being transmitted at child to child level because they involve pleasurable activity. The diagrammatical representation of both the overt and the covert messages can be seen in Figure 3.20.

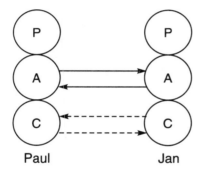

Figure 3.20
A typical ulterior transaction with double meaning message

In this particular type of ulterior transaction, four ego states are at play instead of the usual two. There are also two sets of transactions.

The first one is overt and on a more social level. The adult to adult interaction (i.e.) the stimulus: Would you like to come and see my etchings? and the response: I'd like that very much.

The second message is a covert one and on a more psychological level and the covert message could be interpreted as,

Stimulus
Overt: Would you like to come and see my etchings (with an
          ulterior motive)?
Covert: Would you like to make love?

Response
Overt: I'd like that very much (with an ulterior motive)
Covert: Yes, what a wonderful idea.

This type of interaction is called a duplex ulterior transaction and Berne (1964) said that this type of transaction is common in flirtation games.

Angular transaction

Another type of ulterior transaction is called 'Angular'. Here three ego states are involved. Consider the following interaction between a salesperson and a customer.

> Salesperson: . . . and here we have the latest top of the range model, very stylish but perhaps you are looking for something less pricey.
> Customer: Oh, definitely not, this is exactly what I am looking for. I can in fact well afford it.

The diagrammatical representation of this type of transaction can be seen in Figure 3.21.

Figure 3.21
A typical angular transaction

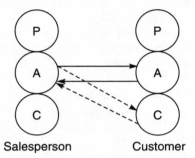

The overt or social level of communication seems to suggest that the salesperson's Adult ego state is addressing the customer's Adult ego state. The covert or psychological level shows that the salesperson's Adult is hooking the customer's Child into buying the product. The customer, not wishing to be outdone, responded by agreeing to buy the product. The salesperson is clearly playing a psychological game where he or she basically dictates the rules. Psychological games are always at play during either a duplex or an angular transaction.

Games analysis

Berne described a psychological game as a series of repetitious and overtly complimentary transactions the true nature of which is ulterior, and leads to a well defined and predictable outcome. The two main characteristics of a psychological game are:

1   Ulterior in nature
2   There is a payoff

By nature, games are always dishonest and have dramatic endings. The person who is playing a game does so to win. Berne stated that for some individuals games are urgently necessary for the maintenance of their health. The implication is that those people will become ill if they do not have the opportunity to engage in games. In a way this is not that difficult to imagine. If for example you are involved in a game-like argument with another person and this person does not want to get involved and retreats with something like, 'I'll let you win', you may in a way feel cheated of that heated argument. This is usually the case when you have prepared yourself a solid case and then as soon as you approach the other person, you get five or six apologies in a row to indicate that it was their mistake. This kind of interaction in fact renders the game player powerless.

People basically learn to play games right from an early age during their interaction with the environment. Can you recall the times you have pretended to be ill so as to avoid going to school? This kind of scenario would be seen as classic example of game playing, although in this context with no serious harm.

Reflect on your 'good young days' when for one reason or another you were engaged in such games as 'mum, my tummy is hurting' so as to avoid, say, eating your mash potato.

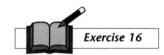

Exercise 16

There are three stages in a game and these are:

- First Degree Game. This is a type of game where it is socially acceptable amongst those concerned
- Second Degree Game. Here there is no permanent damage and the players would prefer to keep it away from the public
- Third Degree Game. This is very serious in terms of intensity and it usually results in one or more players ending up in either courtroom, hospital or mortuary

Some of the psychological games which Berne identified include:

- Kick Me. This is as if I walk around with a big sign on my back, asking others to treat me like a 'mug' and when they do, I complain 'why does this always happen to me?'

Reflect on and note as many Kick Me's scenarios as possible.

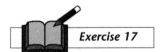

Exercise 17

- Now I've Got You Son Of a Bitch. This is a kind of game where a person knows full well that others are at his or her mercy. Others have little choices but to do as NIGYSOB player wishes. There is with this type of game a sentiment of blackmail.

Reflect on and note as many NIGYSOB scenarios as possible.

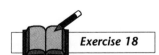

Exercise 18

- See What You Made Me Do. This is where I blame others for a mistake which I made.

Reflect on and note as many SWYMD scenarios as possible.

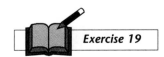

Exercise 19

- Why Don't You – Yes But. This is one of the most commonest game in the literature of games. The following example will demonstrate its basic principle:

Student: 'I find this game concept difficult to understand'
Lecturer: 'Why don't you start with this simple exercise?'
Student: 'Yes, but I find it too childish'
Lecturer: 'Why don't you read a bit more on that subject?'
Student: 'Yes, but every time I do that I get more confused'

This is as if you have an answer to everything I say and yet you give the impression that you want someone to help you.

- RAPO. Simply put this means that the goods are on display, but you cannot have them. It is one of the sexual games which some people engage in. Teasing someone into believing that he or she stands a chance of sexual intercourse, when in fact we do not have the slightest intention of doing so. RAPO is a very good example of the progression of a game from first degree to third degree.

First degree game

At a party and I note that a woman keeps looking in my direction. I acknowledge her non-verbally and give her the impression that I am interested in her. As soon as I have her hooked on to me, I end the game by letting her know that I am not interested in her. I can make this as long or as short as I wish. At the end of the day, I am in total control.

Second degree game

Continuing with the above scenario, my primary gratification in a second degree game comes from rejecting the woman. So what I do is to commit myself seriously but without full commitment. Basically I do not have the slightest intention of making this into a relationship.

Third degree game

Here the situation becomes much more serious and I lead the woman into compromising physical contact and then claim that I have been sexually harassed. I could even make the woman feel worse by enjoying sexual intercourse with her and then say that I was forced into this situation and did so without consenting. The possible outcome of this scenario could be:

1   The woman could go home and kill herself
2   She could kill me
3   Both could fight it out in a courtroom. (Michael Douglas and Demi Moore's film 'Disclosure' has a sentiment of RAPO game in it)

Please refer to Eric Berne's book entitled, *Games People Play, the Psychology of Relationships*, in which he identified numerous psychological games under the headings of, Life Games, Marital Games, Party Games, Sexual Games, Underworld Games, Consulting Room Games and Good Games.

Good games and bad games

By definition, a game suggests an element of ulterior motive, where one person is the winner and the other is the loser. Having said that there are what Berne called 'good games'. 'A good game would be one which contributes both to the well-being of the other players and to the unfolding of the one who is "it"' (Berne, 1964, p.143). One example of such game is the 'Happy to Help Game'. In this situation I am happy to help others and my ulterior motive is that I am making up for my past wickedness. So here we have a situation whereby in the process of satisfying my own needs I help others. Unfortunately there are not many of those types of game.

Berne's concept of transactional analysis is quite extraordinary in that it visually demonstrates the dynamics of communication. We know for example which ego stages we are functioning from and what reactions we get as a result. This offers an individual an opportunity to be fairly calculated in the way he or she interacts with others. Transactional analysis allows people the opportunity to evaluate their transactions and they can if they so wish, change what they say or do. They may also be in a position to use both their cognitive and affective functions in balance with each other rather than using one at the expense of the other.

Script analysis

A script is seen as a blueprint of a person's life map. This basically shows the structure of the person's life from birth to death. James and Jongeward state that a script is like a dramatic stage production, that an individual feels obliged to act out. Script is linked with some early decisions and the position which we take as children. 'It is in the Child ego state and is "written" through the transactions between parents and their child' (James and Jongeward, 1971, p.38). The implication here is that early in life the child takes a certain position which he could play for the rest of his life, for example, 'I am thick', 'I am a loser'. Try Exercise 20.

Draw your life map from birth to the here and now, identify most of the things that have happened.

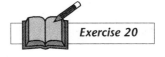

Exercise 20

The above exercise may offer you an idea of the type of script you have. There are essentially three types of scripts and these are as follows.

Productive script suggests that people have an element of control over their lives and can within limits, do what they want. The factor which is believed to contribute to a productive script is acquiring positive strokes. This could be seen as a healthy script to have.

Productive script

In a non-productive script nothing much happens and this is because the person's positive strokes balance out their negative strokes.

Non-productive script

A destructive script leads to destructive behaviour and this may be because of acquiring mainly negative strokes.

Destructive script

Both the non-productive and destructive scripts have what could be described as elements of maladaptiveness within them and as a result can take the form of anyone of the following:

- Never Script. This is like I never get what I really wanted
- Always Script. Here I am stuck in the same groove and I am always doing the same or similar things

- Until or Before Script. I must earn my reward. There is an element here of checking 'what's in it for me' before I take on anything
- After Script. This particular life script implies that there will be trouble after I reach a particular milestone
- Almost Script. I am nearly there but I never quite make it
- Open-Ended Script. I know what I am suppose to do up to a point in time but I have no idea what to do after

According to James and Jongeward (1971) a person's script will always be based on three questions:

- Who am I?
- What am I doing here?
- Who are all those others?

The person could come to any sort of conclusion and whichever he decides, this will reflect the environment and the messages he was brought up with. According to James and Jongeward (1971), infants behave as if they have a radar and they begin to pick up messages about themselves and their worth through their first experiences of being touched or being ignored by others. The messages which those children who are cuddled, and touched affectionately receive are qualitatively different from those received by children who are handled with fright, hostility and anxiety. There is an abundance of script messages which children grow up with, some of the positive ones include:

Positive script messages

- You'll make it one day
- You'll go somewhere
- You'll become somebody
- You are a lovely person
- You are intelligent
- You've always been good at everything
- You've got the gift

Negative script messages

Some of the negative messages are:

- Nothing but trouble since you were born
- No peace when you are around
- Sometimes I wonder where your brain is
- Good for nothing
- You'll never make it

Parents may not be aware of how much of these messages are taken on board by children, nevertheless they make tremendous impressions on children. Having said that, it is interesting to note Perls' remark as quoted by James and Jongeward (1971, p.84), 'As you know, parents are never right. They are either too large or too small, too smart or too dumb. If they are stern, they should be soft, and so on. But when do you find parents who are all right?'

Permissions and injunctions

In order that children may develop their true potential, they need certain permissions in the form of verbal or non-verbal acknowledgements and approvals from their parents. If permissions are not obvious they then pick up messages of injunctions. There are at least eight permissions which are critical for a child's growth and development. Every one of those eight permissions has a counter-permission, which basically inhibit one's growth and development.

Permission to exist – children pick up messages from their parents or significant others early on in their lives to give them an idea as to whether they are wanted or not. Sometimes they may pick up messages to indicate that they are a burden to their parents, in which case this becomes an injunction. Sometimes parents may in a moment of frustration make such statement like, 'Go and play on the motorway'. This would instil the sentiment of 'I wish you were dead'. With these types of messages, children grow up with the idea that their parents would have been better off without them, as a result, they are not motivated to grow and develop.

Permission to be

Permission to feel, as in sensations. Here children ask for permissions to feel and if this is not granted, they then pick up the injunction of 'don't feel'.

Permission to feel

Permission to feel emotion – children ask permission to feel their true emotions, sometimes however they pick up messages to suggest that they should not feel, better still they should not show their true feelings.

Permission to have emotions

Permission to think – sometimes children pick up messages to indicate that they are not allowed to think. 'I'll tell you when to think', 'You only think when I tell you to', 'Don't argue with me boy', and other such messages indicate the element of 'Don't think' injunction.

Permission to think

Permission to be emotionally and physically closer to others – sometimes this is made very obvious to children. Parents say things like 'keep away from that boy or girl,' the child will pick up messages of 'Don't be close'. The sentiment of this particular injunction suggests that one should keep oneself to oneself.

Permission to be close to others physically and emotionally

Permission to be yourself – here children seek permission to be who they are, but if they pick up messages to indicate 'Don't be yourself', they may behave according to how their parents want them to. This is not dissimilar to Rogers' concept of introjection, that is, putting one's feelings and attitudes on hold and taking on the feelings and attitudes of one's parents.

Permission to be yourself

Permission to be whatever age children are – the injunction which they sometimes pick up is reflected in the following: 'Don't be a child' or 'Don't grow up'.

Permission to be whatever age you want to be
Permission to succeed

Permission to succeed – the implication here is that children have to seek permission to succeed in life, but sometimes they pick up messages to indicate that their parents do not really want them to succeed. Some of the possible reasons may be that they do not want their children to be more successful than them or that they would not like their children to be so successful that they may have to move away from home. The injunction therefore is one of 'Don't make it'.

The concept of drivers

Drivers are basically messages which children pick up during their growth and development and these messages eventually become part and parcel of the way they live their scripts. One could say that drivers are the motivating forces behind some of people's behaviour. According to Stewart and Joines (1987), Taibi Kahler identified five of these drivers and these are:

- Be perfect
- Please others
- Try hard
- Be strong
- Hurry up

Be perfect

The implication of the 'Be perfect' driver is that the individual comes to believe that the only way he or she is going to be good enough is if he or she does things to the utmost perfection. 'Be perfect' driver can be seen in the way the individual behaves, for example through speech, tone of voice, gestures, postures and facial expressions. The sentiment of 'You are only good enough if you are perfect' would have been drilled into the individual right from an early age so that he or she comes to believe that this is how it is, and thus develops into a grown-up who always strives for perfection. This kind of behaviour obviously, will eventually lead to mental health problems. However one could guard against such a driver by restructuring one's thinking process by making use of such counter-drivers as 'I am good enough as I am'.

Please others

The 'Please others' driver carries the sentiment that the only way 'I will feel that I am good enough' is if I please others. Therefore I try to please others all the time. This may even include doing things which do not fit in with me. I may for example say that I like some things when in fact I cannot stand them and all this is my attempt to make others happy. The counter-driver to 'Please others' is 'Please yourself' or 'Be selfish sometimes' and this would be a recipe for achieving a healthy mental state.

Try hard

The emphasis of the 'Try hard' driver is that in order to be good enough I have to try hard. Some have described this particular driver as a loser's driver and the implication is that there is always an element of 'just about to but never quite make it'. The counter-driver to the 'Try hard' driver is 'Just do it' and you'll be good enough anyway.

Be strong

The driver 'Be strong' implies that the only way I will be good enough is if I hide my feelings from others. Showing one's feeling is interpreted as weak and this message would have been made clear during a person's early developmental years. The counter-driver is 'Show your feelings'.

Hurry up

The message of this particular driver could be something like, 'the only way I'll be good enough is if I hurry up'. There will most likely be an element of 'hurrying' in what the person does. The counter-driver to the 'Hurry up' driver is 'Take your time' or 'Work to your pace' and you'll be just as good.

Transactional analysis and care delivery

As a theory which explains most if not all forms of communication it helps the carer to make purposeful interventions so that the client can benefit. One could argue that communication underpins caring and this is validated by patients themselves. As a theory of personality, transactional analysis attempts to explain the internal dynamics of the individual. It would seem to be quite logical to presume that if the carers understand how people function, they will be in a better position to help.

It can be deduced that if patients are in crossed transactions with the carer, communication will be hindered. This knowledge will help the latter to try and convert the crossed into complimentary transactions, because this would seem to be the only route through which therapeutic care can be delivered. The same can be said for ulterior transactions, carers would always need to address the client's adult ego state in order to initiate a clear adult response. Knowledge of the ego states will help to confirm this. The reader is invited to undertake the following exercises.

1   Consider the concept of exclusion and its possible effects on behaviour
2   Consider the concept of contamination and its possible effects on behaviour
3   Consider symbiosis (see page 168) and its possible effects on behaviour. Here carers may prevent patients/clients from depending on them and vice versa.

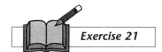

Exercise 21

The effect of positive strokes, negative strokes and the use of touch (for self-concept) can play a crucial role in caring. This can be linked with some of the assumptions of TA, such as, people are okay. These assumptions can serve as a philosophical belief which underpins and dictates future care. The implications of transactional analysis are discussed further in the last chapter which deals with reflection. The therapeutic value of transactional analysis in health care delivery cannot be underestimated. Transactional analysis, through reflection, allows an individual the opportunity to examine the content and structure of his/her communication and by so doing it serves as a tool for enhancing one's self-awareness. Furthermore it provides an individual the opportunity to create a balance between his/her affective and cognitive behaviour. Cognitive behaviour is the theme for the next chapter.

References

Berne, E. (1961). *Transactional Analysis in Psychotherapy. The Classic Handbook To Its Principles*. New York: Grove Press, Inc.

Berne, E. (1964). *Games People Play; The Psychology of Human Relationships*. London: Penguin Books.

Dusay, J.M. and Dusay, K. (1989). 'Transactional analysis.' In: Corsini, R.J. and Wedding, D. (Eds) *Current Psychotherapies*. Itasca, Ill, USA:F.E. Peacock Publishers, Inc.

James, M. and Jongeward, D. (1971). *Born To Win*. New York: Addison-Wesley.

Stewart, I. and Joines, V. (1987). *TA Today. A New Introduction to Transactional Analysis*. Nottingham: Lifespace.

Cognitive development 4

Objectives

After reading this chapter you should be able to:

1 List some of the topics which form part of cognitive psychology
2 Explain the terms: schema, assimilation, accommodation, and adaptation
3 Discuss the notion of irrational thinking
4 Describe Piaget's stages of cognitive development
5 Explain the terms: insight learning, object permanence, egocentricity and concept of conservation
6 Discuss Piaget's notion of moral reasoning
7 Discuss Kohlberg's concept of moral development

The realm of cognitive psychology

One of the factors which is significantly relevant to an individual's internal responses is thought. It could be argued that a person's thought influences the way he or she behaves. Other factors which are linked with thought, include memory, past experiences, attention and ability to solve problems. These factors come under the realm of cognitive psychology. As cognitive psychology is a very broad area, the intention here is to focus on thoughts from Piaget's point of view. It seems logical also to discuss some of Kohlberg's work since it deals with moral reasoning and moral development.

Thoughts can be defined as ways of processing information which are related to a particular time, person or object. Wade and Tavris (1993) define thinking as the mental manipulation of information, and this includes the manipulation of internal representations of objects and situations.

Piaget (1896–1980) and cognitive development

According to Piaget (1952), the origin of thoughts and intellectual processes rest with the concepts of

1 Schema
2 Assimilation

3   Accommodation and

4   Adaptation

Schema can be defined as a cognitive map for processing information. It is also seen as a mould. Hjelle and Ziegler (1992) define schema as an organised structure of knowledge about a particular object, concept, or sequence of events. People therefore behave according to their schema of the world. The word schema has its origin in the work of Edward Tolman (1948) who believed that his experimental rats had developed a mental representation of the maze. Tolman's experiment involved three groups of hungry rats (reward control group, nonreward control group and experimental group), which were trained in a complex maze (see Figure 4.1). One trial took place each day and these three groups of rats were treated as follows. Reward control group rats were always rewarded after each trial, as food was always present in the end box. Nonreward control group rats were not rewarded at all. The experimental group rats were not rewarded for the first 10 days, then on the 11th day they were rewarded (food in the end box). The result showed that on the 12th day the experimental group performed as well as the reward control group. Tolman concluded that for this to happen, the experimental rats must have developed an internal representation of the maze during the first few days before food was introduced, but had no reason to show it until the time when food was in the end box. This is called latent (hidden) learning. This means that the skill is learnt but only demonstrated when it was felt appropriate to do so.

Figure 4.1

Shows a typical illustration of Tolman's experimental maze

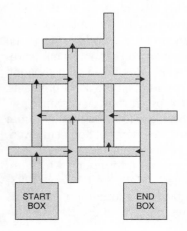

People's thinking process regarding something will depend on their schemata (plural of schema) of that particular thing. If for example my schema of a nurse is that 'she is an angel,' then all my thoughts and expectations of a nurse will be of an angelic woman, not as a man nor as a person with his or her own needs. Piaget (1975) believed that the formation of one's schema (or reformulating one's existing schema) involved a process which includes assimilation, accommodation and adaptation. Consider the schema of a nurse as an angel, others would believe that I have a faulty schema or the wrong idea of who a nurse is. The dynamic interactions between assimilation, accommodation and adaptation would be as follows.

I obtain new information to show me that a man can also be a nurse, I then take in this information. The act of taking in new information is called assimilation. 'Assimilation occurs when there is some kind of cognitive structuring of an external object or event in accordance with the individual's pre-existing cognitive organisation,' Inhelder and Piaget (1958, p.232). Having taken in this new information one now needs to make room in one's existing schema to fit it in. The act of making room to allow for new information is called accommodation. This would mean that I have taken in the idea that a nurse can be either a man or a woman; now I have a different schema of a nurse. As Piaget said, accommodation occurs when the cognitive organisation is modified by the need to deal accurately with the requirements of environmental events. The whole process of assimilation and accommodation is called adaptation. Piaget stated that true adaptation occurs as a result of an equilibrium between assimilation and accommodation. Having said that, assimilation can take place without accommodation, in which case reality is for the individual what he or she wants to believe it is. This may be a possible explanation for people who exhibit symptoms of hallucination. When accommodation occurs without assimilation, one tends to imitate what others do. This is like copying or imitating a behaviour without internalisation.

Assimilation

Accommodation

Adaptation

According to Piaget, the development of intelligence is the highest form of adaptation the child can make with his environment. In this sense schema and adaptation are the two most important concepts in thought processing. One can sometimes have the wrong schema of things, for example one's thoughts and ideas could be different to others. Try Exercise 21.

Write down what you think of the following

- Doctors
- Nurses
- Patients

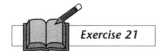

Exercise 21

Discuss this with a colleague or friend and establish any similarities and differences in your ideas.

Identify those positive and negative thoughts. Having done so, now question some of your answers. See if you have any of what would be described as irrational thoughts. This, you may think, is tricky. 'How would I know that my thoughts are irrational?' Consider the following statements:

The world is against me
I am never lucky
Everyone is better off than me
I'll never make it
Everyone is much more intelligent than me
Everyone seems more confident than me

No one fancies me
Why does this always happen to me
I'm always in the wrong queue
Trust me to pick the slowest lane on the motorway

If you have had, at any time, any one of these thoughts, then I would say you have had an irrational thought.

Below are more examples of what one would consider to be irrational thinking.

Irrational thinking

- Nursing is about caring for poorly people
- Nursing takes place in hospitals
- Nurses are angels
- Nurses have to be submissive to be able to care
- Nurses are handmaidens to doctors
- Nurses should not ask for more money
- Patients are passive recipients of care
- Doctors are here to prescribe medicine
- Doctors have easy lives
- Doctors are to be obeyed
- Patients come first

OK-ness concept

Let us explore what you truly think of yourself and of others. In an attempt to enable you to self reflect, Thomas Harris's (1973) model of the four life positions are used. These are:

- I'm not OK – You're OK
- I'm not OK – You're not OK
- I'm OK – You're not OK
- I'm OK – You're OK

A simplistic explanation of the 'OK-ness' concept is as follows, OK is good and Not OK can be either bad or feeling inferior.

Harris (1973) believes that each person occupies these four life positions and by the time a child reaches the age of 2 years, he or she has already decided on the first three positions. Roughly translated therefore the child comes to the conclusion that

- He or she is inferior to others
- Everyone is bad
- He or she is superior to others

Please note here that feeling is substituted for thought. Harris's original writings refer to 'OK-ness feeling'. One could argue that there is an inter-action between feeling and thinking, for example I have this 'not OK-ness feeling', I therefore conclude that I am either bad or inferior. For this to happen I would have had to mentally process or manipulate the incoming information. Hence the reason for the substitution. Harris argues that the child becomes fixated at the 'I'm not OK you're OK life position'. This becomes more or less permanent. The child can move to the second and third life positions depending on his or her interaction with significant others. One could say that even as adults, at any time during people's life, they will go through all these life positions. Consider Exercise 22.

Reflect on yourself and see if you can think of situations when you thought that
You are inferior to others
The whole human race is bad
You are superior to others
There is goodness in everyone
You could do a job better than someone else

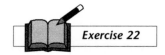

Exercise 22

Having done that, if you feel brave enough to discuss these with someone else (friend, colleague or partner), feel free to do so. If not, reflecting on these situations would have served a good purpose.

Harris believes that the first three positions (I'm not OK – You're OK, I'm not OK – You're not OK, I'm OK – You're not OK) are unconscious.

Reflect on some of your thoughts and list them under the headings of Pessimistic Thoughts and Optimistic Thoughts.

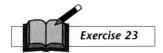

Exercise 23

Explore your list of pessimistic thoughts and analyse these in an attempt to identify some of the rationales as to why you think the way you do. You may well find that one of the contributory factors is the way you have been brought up.

Piaget's stages of cognitive development

Piaget suggested that an individual's thoughts change throughout development in a systematic way. According to Piaget, there are four major stages of cognitive development and these are

1   Sensorimotor stage (birth to approximately 2 years)
2   Pre-operational stage (from 2 to 7 years)
3   Concrete operational stage (from 7 to 11/12 years)
4   Formal Operational Stage (from 12 years onward)

Piaget's sentiment seems to suggest that the dynamism between assimilation, accommodation, adaptation leads to the construction of a complex system of 'action-schemes and organising reality in terms of spatio-temporal and causal structures' Piaget and Inhelder (1969, p.4). Children do this through their perceptions and movements, hence sensorimotor. This period emphasises the reflexes of the infant and in particular the sucking and palmar reflexes. The infant's actions start from being accidental to being much more controlled and calculated. Here the infant is able to establish the relationships between actions and consequences. The infant learns from unintentional behaviour and prolongs or repeats interesting

Sensorimotor period

acts. If for example an object, which is outside the reach of an infant, is placed on a rug and the infant causes the object to move by accidentally pulling on the rug, the infant will establish the connection between the rug and the object, so the infant will come to learn that if he or she pulls the rug he or she will be able to reach and grasp the object. In this sense the infant's behaviour becomes increasingly intentional. Gradually however, the child will come to develop a 'sudden comprehension or insight'. That is being able to suddenly find the solution to a problem. Insight learning was studied by Wolfgang Kohler (1925), with the help of his chimpanzee Sultan. Kohler's experiment involved placing some sort of fruit beyond Sultan's reach, outside the cage and placing some bamboo sticks nearby. The bamboo sticks on their own were not long enough to reach the fruit. After many unsuccessful attempts at reaching for the fruit, Sultan suddenly, as if in a flash of inspiration, started to fit the bamboo sticks together and used them to rake in the fruit. Kohler concluded that Sultan was able to formulate the relationships between the sticks and achieving his goal.

Kohler and insight learning

Object permanence

Piaget argued that during this period, the infant develops the concept of object permanence, and this basically means that the infant develops an awareness that an object continues to exist even when it cannot be perceived. 'At about five to seven months, when the child is about to seize an object and you cover it with a cloth or move it behind a screen, the child simply withdraws his already extended hand or in the case of an object of special interest (his bottle, for example), begins to cry or scream with disappointment. He reacts, therefore, as if the object had been reabsorbed' (Piaget and Inhelder, 1969, p.14). There is an element of 'out of sight, out of mind' in the behaviour of the infant of that particular age group.

The pre-operational level

During the sensorimotor period, true thought as such is not apparent. According to Piaget, the ability to form a mental representation about any object or event, sees the beginning of the pre-operational period of cognitive development. Here symbols and language are used to represent things. Piaget's argument is that during this period children may be able to think, but they do not have the mental ability to reason. These children also show what is described as the concept of egocentrism or egocentricity. This means that children have a tendency to see things only from their own perspectives. One could argue that at times egocentrism is obvious even in the behaviour of adults. I have noticed on more than one occasion that my adult students, on the last day before their holidays, would wish me a nice holiday, even though, it was they themselves who were going on holidays and not me. One can only conclude from this that they must have thought that whenever they are on holiday, I too am on holiday.

Egocentricity

Conservation

Another feature of the pre-operational child is the latter's ability to grasp the concept of conservation. Conservation means that the physical properties (amount, size, volume, and weight) of things remain the same even though their shapes or appearances may change.

The concrete operational period

According to Piaget, this period means that the child has captured the concept of conservation and is now less egocentric. This demonstrates that the child has developed a higher level of intellectual achievement and the capacity for adult logic thinking. This logic thinking however, is confined to concrete rather than abstract ideas. The concrete operational child can now focus on more than one dimensions of a problem. There is also an element of subjectivity in the child's moral judgements.

Piaget argued that by the time these individuals reach the formal operational period, these adolescents can think more or less like adults. They are able to solve problems mentally and deal in abstract terms. Logic becomes a possible tool of thought. The thinking of these individuals show distinct characteristics and some of these include

The formal operational period

1   They can work with an hypothetical concept
2   They show deductive ability
3   They can use inferences to arrive at conclusions
4   They can generate and test hypotheses

Piaget used his 'Pendulum Problem' to demonstrate the development of the individual's powers of reasoning, deduction and inferences. Presented with a pendulum, a weight swinging from a string, the individual is asked which factors determine the speed of the pendulum's swing. Piaget stated that the pendulum can be made to swing faster or slower by varying the length of the string. The differences in the weight attached do not affect the rate of oscillation, neither does the height from which it is dropped nor the initial force used for the first swing. Piaget found that subjects at the level of concrete operations varied everything at the same time and were convinced that varying the weight had an effect. The pre-adolescents who would be at the formal operational stage, found that there was no link between the various weights and the rate of oscillation, so they would exclude the weights.

Piaget and moral reasoning

Piaget introduced the concept of moral realism to imply that one's obligations and values are determined by the law or the order itself, independent of intentions and relationships. Piaget argued that moral realism leads to objective responsibility, for example one would evaluate an act in terms of the degree to which it falls within the boundaries of the law rather than whether one has malicious intent of violating the law. Piaget's classic example is the story of the boy who broke a tea cup while trying to steal some jam and another boy who accidentally broke a whole tray full of tea cups. When children of the pre-operational period are asked to say who was the naughtiest boy, they would reply, the boy who broke a tray full of cups. The development of moral reasoning starts right from an early age through the process of socialisation. Having said that, children do not necessarily have to understand the concept of values before developing some sort of moral reasoning. They believe however, that if they were to violate some moral rules, they would be punished, as Atkinson et al. (1994, p.84) put it, 'God would punish them or they would be hit by a car'.

Kohlberg (born 1927) and moral development

Kohlberg (1984) believes that the foundation of moral development is found in an individual's level of reasoning. The major developmental stages of reasoning include

- intuitive
- concrete operational
- formal operational

Kohlberg argues that a parallel can be drawn between an individual's logic and moral stage. For example an individual who is at a low level of reasoning will be at a low moral stage and similarly a high level of reasoning could lead to a high moral stage. 'To act in a morally high way requires a high stage of moral reasoning. One cannot follow moral principles. . . if one does not understand or believe in them' (Kohlberg, 1984, p.172).

Kohlberg extended the work of Piaget and came up with a six-stage model of moral development. Kohlberg's studies involved setting his subjects some moral dilemmas to which they have to provide answers with rationales. One such typical dilemma is 'The Heinz Dilemma'.

The Heinz dilemma

'In Europe, a woman was near death from a very bad disease, a special kind of cancer. There was one drug that the doctors thought might save her. It was a form of radium that a druggist in the same town had recently discovered. The drug was expensive to make, but the druggist was charging 10 times what the drug cost him to make. He paid $200 for the radium and charged $2000 for a small dose of the drug. The sick woman's husband, Heinz, went to everyone he knew to borrow the money, but he could get together only about $1000, which was half what it was cost. He told the druggist that his wife was dying and asked him to sell it cheaper or let him pay later. But the druggist said, "No, I discovered the drug and I'm going to make money from it." Heinz got desperate and broke into the man's store to steal the drug for his wife' (Kohlberg, 1981, p.12).

In one such investigation, Kohlberg studied 75 American boys from early adolescence onward. From these types of studies Kohlberg was able to construct what he described as a typology of definite and universal levels of development in moral thought. This typology has three distinct levels of moral thinking, preconventional, conventional and post-conventional and each of these levels have two stages (see Figure 4.2).

Preconventional level

According to Kohlberg, the child responds to cultural rules and the ideas of good and bad, right or wrong. These are interpreted in terms of their consequences (i.e.) punishment, reward, or exchange of favours. This level is reached by most children under 9 years of age, some adolescents, and many adolescents and adult criminal offenders.

Stage 1: The punishment and obedience orientation

In the punishment and obedience stage the physical consequences of the action dictate whether the action is good or bad, value and human meaning are important. There is here an element of obeying the rules to escape punishment. This is seen purely from an egocentric point of view.

A child at the instrumental relativist orientation stage tends to focus on action which leads to rewards. Therefore rules are followed when 'there is something in it for me'. Right is seen as what is fair.

Stage 2: The instrumental relativist orientation

Kohlberg (1984) states that this level of morality emphasises maintaining the expectations of one's family, groups, or nation as being valuable in its own right. Consequences of action are not relevant. There is also an element of loyalty to the order. This level is reached by most adolescents and adults.

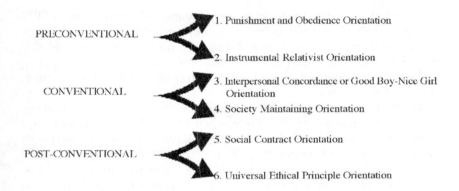

PRECONVENTIONAL
1. Punishment and Obedience Orientation
2. Instrumental Relativist Orientation

CONVENTIONAL
3. Interpersonal Concordance or Good Boy-Nice Girl Orientation
4. Society Maintaining Orientation

POST-CONVENTIONAL
5. Social Contract Orientation
6. Universal Ethical Principle Orientation

Figure 4.2
Kohlberg's (1984) stages of moral development

Conventional level

The whole sentiment of the interpersonal concordance or 'Good boy' 'Nice girl' orientation stage is that behaviour is based on condition of worth, for example good behaviours are those behaviours which please and are approved by others. As Kohlberg said, 'behaviour is frequently judged by intention – the judgement "he means well" becomes important for the first time' (Kohlberg, 1981, Vol.1, p.18).

Stage 3: The interpersonal concordance

In this, the society maintaining orientation stage, 'right' is interpreted according to the law of society. The focus therefore is on doing one's duty, showing respect for authority, and maintaining the given social order for its own sake.

Stage 4: The society maintaining orientation

Post-conventional, autonomous, or principled level

Kohlberg argues that there is a clear effort to define moral values and principles which have validity and are applicable on a global perspective. That is separate from 'the authority of the groups or people holding these principles and apart from the individual's own identification with these groups' (Kohlberg, 1981, Vol. 1, p.18). A minority of adults reach this level and only after the age of 20 years.

The sentiment reflected by the social contract orientation suggests that what is right tends to be defined according to both the welfare of society and in terms of life being a universal human right.

Stage 5: The social contract orientation

Stage 6: The universal ethical principle orientation

The universal ethical principle orientation is seen as the highest level of morality because it focuses on the equality of human rights. People's dignity is respected.

The two main themes which Kohlberg focused on during his analysis of the answers to the moral dilemmas which he set his subjects, were:

1   Why do people obey, what were their moral actions?
2   What value do they have of human life?

Running the subjects' action parallel to the value they placed on human life, Kohlberg's conclusion is shown in Table 1.

Kohlberg's findings suggest that moral development is sequential, starting with stage 1 and working its way through to stage 6, without skipping steps. The length of time through which children move from one stage to another varies and it is possible for one person to be found half in and half out of a particular stage. Moral reasoning of stages 3 and 4 does not occur before stages 1 and 2.

Perhaps one of the most important question here is, 'do one's thoughts and morals influence the way one delivers care?' The answer would be a categorical 'Yes' and perhaps more so if the carer is lacking in self-awareness. Similarly awareness of one's own schema about a particular object or person would enhance person to person interaction. For example an awareness of my own thoughts and the way I feel will enable me to acknowledge other people's points of view. Helpers' moral standards will in many ways dictate the extent of the care they offer. It can also be argued that the helper's knowledge underpins care delivery. The growth and development of knowledge rest with the person's interpretation of his or her world and thus the person's perception. Perception and behaviour are the topics of Chapter 5.

Table 1
Reason for obedience and value imposed on human life. Adapted from Kohlberg (1984, Vol. 1, pp.19–20)

Stages	Motive for moral action	Value of human life
1	Obey rules to avoid punishment	Value of human life is confused with the value of physical objects and is based on the social status or physical attributes of the possessor
2	Conform to obtain rewards	The value of human life is seen as instrumental to the satisfaction of the needs of its possessor or of other people
3	Conform to avoid disapproval	The value of human life is based on the empathy and affection of family members and others towards its possessor
4	Conform to avoid censure by legitimate authorities and resultant guilt	Life is conceived as sacred in terms of its place in a categorical moral or religious order of rights and duties
5	Conform to maintain the respect of the impartial spectator judging in terms of community welfare	Life is valued both in terms of relation to community welfare and in terms of life being a universal human right
6	Conform to avoid self-condemnation	Human life is sacred – a universal human value of respect for the individual

References

Atkinson, R.L., Atkinson, R.C., Smith, E.E. and Bem, D.J. (1994). *Introduction to Psychology*. London: Harcourt Brace College Publishers.

Harris, T.A. (1973). *I'am ok – You're ok*. London and Sydney: Pan Books.

Hjelle, L.A. and Ziegler, D.J. (1992). *Personality Theories. Basic Assumptions, Research, and Applications*. New York: McGraw-Hill International Editions.

Inhelder, B. and Piaget, J. (1958). *The Growth of Logical Thinking from Childhood to Adolescence*. New York: Basic Books; London: Routledge and Kegan Paul.

Kohlberg, L. (1981). *The Psychology of Moral Development. The Nature and Validity of Moral Stages,* Vol. I. San Francisco, CA: Harper and Row.

Kohlberg, L. (1984). *The Philosophy of Moral Development. Essays on Moral Development*, Vol. II. San Francisco, CA: Harper and Row.

Kohler, W. (1925). *The Mentality of Apes*. New York: Harcourt Brace.

Piaget, J. (1952). *The Origins of Intelligence in Children*. New York: International Universities Press.

Piaget, J. (1975). *The Development of Thought Equilibration of Cognitive Structures*. Oxford: Basil Blackwell.

Piaget, J. and Inhelder, B. (1969). *The Psychology of the Child*. London and Henley: Routledge and Kegan Paul.

Tolman, E.C. (1948). 'Cognitive maps in rats and men.' *Psychological Review*, **55**, 189–208.

Wade, C. and Tavris, C. (1993). *Psychology*. New York: Harper Collins College Publishers.

Perception and behaviour 5

Objectives

After reading this chapter you should be able to:

1   Define perception and explain its intra- and interpersonal properties
2   Discuss how perception is structured and categorised
3   Understand why sometimes people may perceive the wrong picture
4   Explain the concept of self-monitoring
5   Discuss perceptual constancy
6   Recognise some of the factors influencing perception
7   Discuss how the helper's perception can influence health care delivery

Perception: an intrapersonal and an interpersonal phenomenon

Epictetus (1st century AD) is quoted to have expressed the sentiment that people are disturbed not so much by the events as by the views they take of them. A modern version is offered by Hastorft *et al.* (1970, p.5) who point out, 'the world is not merely revealed to us; rather, we play an active role in the creation of our experiences'. These beliefs point to the fact that people are directly responsible for what they perceive, but may not always be aware of their own influences. What is also true is that perception is directly influenced by past and present experiences. Perception, like transactional analysis can be explored from both an internal and external perspective, the difficulty however is how to differentiate between the two. Myers and Myers (1992) argue that perception may be considered as an internal process because certain things happen inside people's heads when they perceive. At the same time, this perception is conditioned by the past and present experience of the sociocultural climate people live in.

What is perception?

Perception can simply be described as the interpretation of sensory input. Obviously without sensation it is virtually impossible to perceive. Sensation is the actual reception of any stimulation, which includes all the senses. One's perception is influenced by numerous factors and amongst those, are one's past experience and motivational state. Hastorft *et al.* (1970) include raw feelings as part of one's experience. Raw feelings, are taken to mean those feelings which one has about something or someone that one cannot quite explain. This is similar to what Eric Berne called one's Little Professor. The common usage of raw feeling is 'intuition', for example an individual knows that something is right or wrong but cannot offer any evidence to validate it. I can feel something is wrong with a patient and I do not know what it is. This sentiment is further reinforced when it later transpired that something was indeed wrong with the patient. Intuition is said to play a very important part in the way self perceives others.

The perceptual process is believed to have numerous properties and these include

- structure
- constancy and
- meaningfulness

People are flooded with perceptual stimuli that if they are to process every single one of them, their brain would have difficulty coping. Instead they tend to categorise the incoming stimuli. In order to demonstrate this point, I would like to take you through a similar process to that which, according to Hastorft *et al.* (1970), Leeper (1935) has used. Have a go at Exercise 24.

Step 1: Spend about 1 minute looking at Figure 5.1

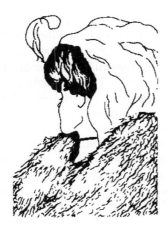

Step 2: Now look at Figure 5.2

What do you see? One guess is that you will most likely see the picture of a young woman. If the picture of an old woman (as seen in Figure 5.3) was shown to you first, then the probability is that you would have seen the picture of an old woman in the ambiguous picture in Figure 5.2. Leeper (1935) showed that 95 per cent of people who were exposed to the picture of the young woman first, saw the young woman first when presented with the second picture which is the ambiguous picture. Similarly 100 per cent

Structure: How do we perceive?

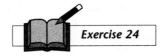

Figure 5.1
This is the sketch portrait of a Young Woman

of those people who were exposed to the picture of the old woman first, reported seeing only the picture of the old woman when presented with the ambiguous picture.

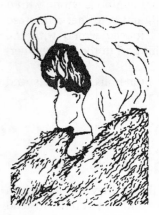

Figure 5.2
This sketch is rather ambiguous

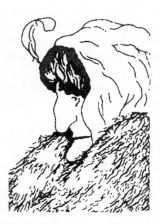

Figure 5.3
This is the sketch portrait of an Old Woman

Categorisational feature of perception

Hastorft *et al.* (1970, p.6) stated, 'one of the most salient features of the person's participation in structuring his experiential world can be described as a categorising process. He extracts stimuli from the world and forces them into a set of categories.' This means that a person tends to view others by pigeon-holing them into different categories, for example one could categorise people by their physical attributes which include their colour, build, height, and even accent. People can also be categorised by their functions and roles. Perhaps some conclusion could be drawn here to suggest that there is a relationship between the way one categorises people and the way one interacts with them.

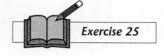

Exercise 25

Self-reflect on some of the categorisations you may have employed in your perception of others and check out if your behaviour was influenced by the particular label you used. Emerging issues can form the basis of a group discussion.

From Figure 5.4, if for example I was to categorise you as an aggressive person, my behaviour is bound to be influenced by my perception of you and this in turn will influence how you behave towards me. Duck's (1997) concept of positive and negative reciprocity would explain people's interpersonal behaviour. The implication is that if you perceive me negatively, it follows that your behaviour will be negative towards me. I in turn will reciprocate both perception and behaviour. The end result is a negative interaction. The same dynamic would apply in a positive reciprocity except in this case perception and behaviour will be positive. 'If we can classify a person according to certain traits or concepts, we can increase

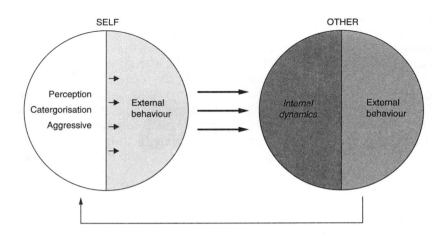

Figure 5.4
Shows the dynamic relationship between perception and external behaviour of self during an interaction with another person

the predictability of our interpersonal world' (Hastorft *et al.*, 1970, p.14). This however does not mean to say that one's prediction will always be right. Two issues emerge here and these are

1   People may perceive the wrong picture
2   People may perceive the right picture, but this may be what others want them to see

Perceiving the wrong picture

Why do people perceive the wrong picture sometimes? As perceivers, people would like to think that their perceptions are always accurate. Unfortunately such a thought can only exist as a delusion. Reality suggests that at one time or another, every single person has perceived a wrong picture. According to Icheiser (1949) cited in Heider (1958, p.57), as the perceivers, people are very important elements in the total situation which 'determines and evokes the type of behaviour the other person is expected to play in the given relation'. The implication here is that one's own presence either evokes or suppresses the way others behave. An example would be that I, as a father, always see my son in the role of son. Similarly my students always see me in the role of teacher. Chances are as health care professionals, we may always see our clients as clients and not as individuals. What we seem to be doing is ascribing a role to people and then observing them in that context. Heider explained this succinctly, 'as if we always carry a flash light with a filter of red colour when examining an empty room; we would then ascribe the colour to the room'. It becomes obvious that in this situation, one is prone to make mistakes, hence one perceives the wrong picture. Other possible explanations as to why an individual misperceives may include egocentric viewing and viewing through the 'eyes of another'.

Egocentric perspective

Egocentric viewing suggests that people perceive the world from their own particular points of view and that they are unable to see it from the points of view of others. According to Piaget (1952), the concept of egocentricity emerges in the pre-operational stage of cognitive development (see Chapter 4). Piaget argued that a child between the age of 2 and 7 years does not possess the ability to see things from the points of view of others. A typical example which reflects a child's egocentric state is captured in the following hypothetical interaction between an adult (Dev) and a child (Darren) in the pre-operational stage.

> Dev: Darren, do you have a brother?
> Darren: Yes
> Dev: What is your brother's name?
> Darren: My brother is called Jason
> Dev: Does Jason have a brother?
> Darren: No

Here Darren knows that he has a brother, but cannot grasp the idea that Jason too has a brother and that he himself is in fact Jason's brother. Although Piaget's concept of egocentricity is the growth and development of children of a certain age, it could be argued that everyone carries around with him or her what could be called the residual effect of egocentrism. For example:

> Teachers see it from teachers' points of view
> Students see it from students' points of view
> Rich people see it from rich people's points of view, similarly
> Poor people see it from poor people's points of view
> Doctors see it from a medical point of view and the list goes on

If when a situation calls for us to see it from the other person's perspective, and we fail to do so then it becomes obvious that we will perceive the wrong picture. Imagine the implication of not being able to develop the skill to empathise with a patient, when the only way empathic understanding can be achieved is by actually being able to see the situation from the patient's perspectives.

Seeing it from the eyes of another

Heider (1958, p.55) argues that misperceptions occur when 'the properties of a person are mediated to us through what other people say or write about him, through gossips, newspapers, etc.' In this case, others would have to interpret their own set of cues, and this may be integrated with false beliefs, which would then be conveyed to us. This would be as if we are seeing the world from their perspectives. When we read a newspaper, we take on what the journalist wants us to know rather than how it really is. Those of us who have played Chinese whispers will know full well the implication of receiving information from a source other than the primary one. There could be an incongruence between the actual event and the journalist's account. Transferring this idea to health care delivery points to the fact that if a patient is described as difficult or non-compliant, then it is most likely that one will be influenced by this category or label. We may dare to say that what we hear from others regarding person 'A' will not make any difference in the way we interact with that person, reality however suggests that what we hear from others, about a particular person, is greatly significant in the way we deal with that person. To know how it really is, one has to be there, experiencing it, and even then the chances are that the true picture may not be entirely what it seems.

People's predictions about others are not always right, and that goes for Mystic Meg as well. Wrong predictions will have serious implications on health care delivery. If I am labelled as a difficult patient, then I will be perceived as a difficult patient. If I am perceived as a hopeless case, then I am treated as a hopeless case. If you perceive me as an invalid, you may then want to do everything for me, thus encouraging me to be dependent on you and so the prophecy goes on. If as professional care-givers we become aware of different labels we are likely to employ when we care for patients or clients, the quality of care that we deliver will improve.

What we see may not necessarily be correct

It would be true to say that sometimes people may want us to perceive what is in fact not true, for example magicians do a pretty good job at dictating and guiding our perceptions. Snyder (1974, p.526) points to the fact that 'although non-verbal behaviour may often escape voluntary attempts at censorship, there have been numerous demonstrations that individuals can voluntarily express various emotions with their vocal and/or facial expressive behaviour in such a way that their expressive behaviour can be accurately interpreted by observers'. This would suggest that it is possible for people to wear the right face for the right time. One would be wrong to think that this is the domain of only professional actors, who are pretty good at presenting themselves as appropriate to the needs of the scene. A brief analysis of the role of politicians, would lead one to conclude that they would see wearing the right face to suit the right environment as a prerequisite to their job. One sees numerous political figures hugging and kissing babies and children, especially when an election is imminent, does this mean that they all love other people's children? Indeed not, in fact some politicians may think of children as 'brats' and their behaviour therefore would be incongruent with their thoughts. Unfortunately one is not in the right place to detect what the true feelings and thoughts of these people are. The implication is that although one may perceive the other person correctly, this does not necessarily mean that one is right. Observers may well be led into perceiving what others want them to see.

The meaningless hugs and kisses

The façade

Why would people behave in a way to deliberately give others the wrong picture? This is an interesting question. Snyder's (1974) sentiment suggests that if for example I learn that my affective experience and expression are socially unacceptable, then I may monitor how I present myself to others. The word monitor is taken to mean observe and control. My rationale for self-monitoring could include any of the following.

- Communicate accurately my true emotional state through an intensified expressive presentation, as in an overexaggerated way
- Communicate accurately a feeling which suits the event or situation, as in professional mourners
- To hide what may be seen as an inappropriate emotional state by appearing vacant and expressionless
- To experience a pseudoemotion because a non-response could be seen as inappropriate

Snyder's concept of self-monitoring

How does one self monitor then? Snyder (1974, p.527) states 'one set of cues for guiding self-monitoring is the emotional expressive behaviour of other similar comparison persons in the same situation'. This basically means that if I am uncertain of how I should react emotionally, then I look to the behaviour of others for guidance, for example if others cry then I cry as well. Self-monitoring is a learned behaviour, perhaps very much like Bandura's (1974) idea of observational learning (see Chapters 8 and 11). Some people are extremely good at self-monitoring, whilst others may not have such well-developed monitoring skills. It is said that for those people, their behaviour will be a true reflection of their feelings and emotions. The picture which is emerging suggests that there are two types of people, those who are high on self-monitoring, that is a person who 'out of a concern for social appropriateness, is particularly sensitive to the expression and self presentation of others in social situations and uses these cues as guidelines for monitoring his own self presentation' (Snyder, 1974, p.528) and those who are low in self-monitoring, and whose behaviour suggests a congruence with their emotions and feelings. Hamachek (1992, pp.24–25) states, 'high self monitors are good "people readers"; they are people who have developed the ability to monitor carefully their own behaviour and to adjust skilfully the self they are presenting when signals from others tell them that they are not having the desired effect. . . . . . Low self monitors, on the other hand seem not so concerned about the social cues that surround them; instead, they tend to express what they feel rather than tailor their presentation of self to fit the situation.'

High and low self monitors

Snyder et al (1983) argue that self-monitoring is a major influence of self-regulated behaviour, for example people who are high in self-monitoring tend to regulate their behaviour according to the immediate situation. This basically means that they observe what is going on and behave accordingly. People who are described as low in self-monitoring tend to behave according to their intrapersonal dynamics. Baron and Byrne (1991) state that low self monitors are more likely to speak in the first person, using I, Me, and My, as compared to high self monitors, who speak in the third person like He, She, They, and so on. High self monitors are also more concerned about what others do and how they themselves react, whereas low self monitors tend to focus on their own behaviour and reactions. Snyder *et al.* (1983) show that high self monitors chose their friends on the basis of their ability in areas of interest to them. Snyder argues that to be such a friend means to be valued for that particular skill. 'Presumably, were your skills to diminish, you would no longer be invited to be an activity partner' (Snyder, 1987, p.67). Low self monitors on the other hand chose their friends according to how much they like them. 'Presumably, as long as you continue to be generally similar and hence well liked, you will be sought out for the pleasure of your company' (Snyder, 1987, p.67).

Do you consider yourself a high or low self monitor?
Do you for example watch what others do, then you behave accordingly?
Or is your behaviour an expression of your true feelings?
Have a go at Exercise 26.

Consider the following statements as your personal reactions to the number of different situations and place a T (for True or Mostly True) or an F (for False or Not Usually True) against each of those items.

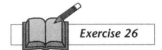

Exercise 26

1 I find it difficult to copy the behaviour of other people
2 My behaviour is usually an expression of my true inner feelings, attitudes and beliefs
3 At parties and social gatherings, I do not attempt to do or say things that others will like
4 I can only argue for ideas which I already believe
5 I can make impromptu speeches even on topics about which I have almost no information
6 I guess I put on a show to entertain or impress people
7 When I am uncertain how to act in a social situation, I look to the behaviour of others for cues
8 I would probably make a good actor
9 I rarely need the advice of my friends to choose movies, books or music
10 I sometimes appear to others to be experiencing deeper emotions than I actually am
11 I laugh more when I watch a comedy with others than when alone
12 In a group of people I am rarely the centre of attention
13 In different situations and with different people, I often act like very different persons
14 I am not particularly good at making other people like me
15 Even if I am not enjoying myself, I often pretend to be having a good time
16 I am not always the person I appear to be

17   I would not change my opinions (or the way I do things) in order to please someone else or win their favour

18   I have considered being an entertainer

19   In order to *get* along and be liked, I tend to be what people expect me to be rather than anything else

20   I have never been good at games like charades or improvisational acting

21   I have trouble changing my behaviour to suit different people and different situations

22   At a party I let others keep the jokes and stories going

23   I feel a bit awkward in company and do not show up quite so well as I should

24   I can look anyone in the eye and tell a lie with a straight face (if for a right end)

25   I may deceive people by being friendly when I really dislike them

The 25-item Self-Monitoring Scale. From *Public Appearances/Private Realities. The Psychology of Self-Monitoring* by Mark Snyder © 1987 by W.H. Freeman and Company. Used with permission.

Whilst it may be true that people can be extremely vigilant in the way they behave, for example they may watch and behave according to the demand of the situation, it would be wrong to believe that the low self monitors always exhibit behaviours which are congruent with how they feel or think at any particular time. One could argue that even with low self monitors, there is an element of 'behaving according to how the situation dictates'. Perhaps this is how it should in fact be. This points to an ideal trait which consists of a mixture between low self monitor and high self monitor because, as Hamachek (1992) says, there are benefits and pitfalls at either extreme (see Figures 5.5 and 5.6).

Figure 5.5

Benefits of low self monitors and pitfalls of high monitors

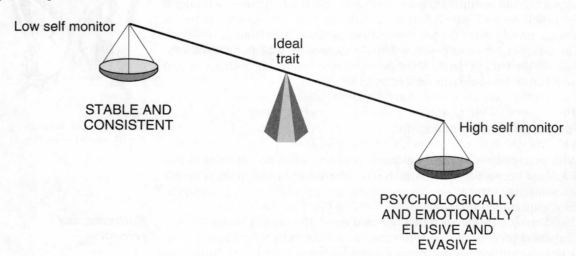

Low self monitor

STABLE AND CONSISTENT

Ideal trait

High self monitor

PSYCHOLOGICALLY AND EMOTIONALLY ELUSIVE AND EVASIVE

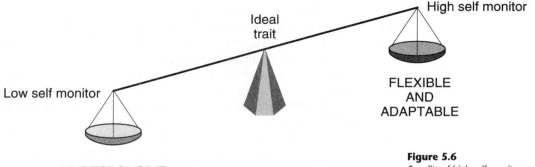

Figure 5.6
Benefits of high self monitors and pitfalls of low self monitors

Perceptual constancy

Perceptual constancy, also known as perceptual stability, can be described as the accurate perception of an object even though the sensory patterns they produce are in a state of change. For example we perceive an aeroplane as an aeroplane whether it is stationary or in flight. When the aeroplane is in flight, although its image on our retina is small we do not perceive it as a small aeroplane. Our perceptual process is able to keep the image of the aeroplane intact in our brain. This particular type of constancy is called size constancy. Other types of constancy include, colour (a red car is a red car whether we look at it in daylight or at night), brightness (snow is perceived as white both at night and during daylight), and location (when we travel at speed, although the image of houses and trees move on our retina, we recognise these objects as stationary).

Size, colour, brightness and location constancy

The perceptual processes are such that they give meaning to our sensory input. Have a look at Figure 5.7. What you will most likely see is a picture of a butterfly and not black patches. This suggests that perception is organised into meaningful units, for example it is much more meaningful for people to see Figure 5.7 as a butterfly than as some black patches. A similar principle is adopted when other people's behaviour is observed. The behaviour of some people will make sense to us, whilst others will confuse us. We tend to ignore those people whose behaviour confuses us and we focus on those we can understand.

Perception is meaningful

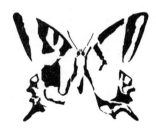

Figure 5.7
Picture of black patches which form the shape of a butterfly

Factors influencing perception

With perception, there is an element of seeing what people want to see. There are numerous factors which may be responsible for making people see what they want to see. Some of these include motivation, past experience, expectation and time.

Can people be deceived by their own eyes? The answer is 'yes'. People can and in fact are deceived on numerous occasions by what they see. This is linked to human factor and one such factor is motivation. Numerous

Motivation and perception

studies have shown that hunger, for example, affects perception. When people are hungry and starving, their most detestable dish appears as cordon bleu. There is a clear implication that whatever drives people at any particular time will have some bearing on how they perceive the events or the situations. Consider the following scenario.

Let us suppose I am a supporter of Manchester United and you support Leeds United. Come the big day, my team is in action against your team. Ten minutes into the match, Leeds United managed to put the ball in Manchester United's goal. The referee however, blew his whistle and called it a no-goal, because one of Leeds United's players was offside. Both you and I want our own team to win, therefore it is most likely that you will argue that your player was not on the offside position, whilst I would be inclined to believe that the referee was right in calling a no-goal. It is obvi-

Right or wrong depends on which side of the fence one happens to be

ous that both of us cannot be right. Having said that, because winning is the name of the game, both of us will continue to believe that we are right and in your case you will be furious at the referee's decision, whereas I will see the referee as having made a good judgement based on his excellent powers of observation.

In the case of the above scenario, it is a question of which side you are on. People are motivated by what interests them. Most advertisers have got us figured out in the sense that they know what is an attention 'getter', sex therefore is used as an instrument to attract our attention.

Past experience

Chance (1989, p.26) argues, 'past learnning also affects our vision. For instance, the chances are good that you did not notice the typographical error in the previous sentence. People regularly see words spelled correctly when in fact they are not.' Perhaps the role of past experience can be demonstrated through Exercise 27.

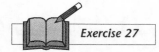

Exercise 27

Have a look at these two cards below.

Show these cards for a brief moment to a colleague and ask him or her to identify them. It is most likely that the answer will only be half correct. This is to do with people's past experience of the nature of playing cards. Cards as we know them do not have two distinct halves. So a quick glance at the above cards will usually lead us to identify them according to where our focus happens to be aimed at. For example if we focus on the top half of the card in Figure 5.8(a), we will see nine of Clubs, we will then presume that the whole card is a nine of Clubs card. Similarly if we focus on the bottom half of the card, we will see nine of Spades, here again we will presume that the whole card is a nine of Spades card. The same phenomenon will apply to the card in Figure 5.8(b).

Based on the principle of the above phenomenon, it could be argued that people's behaviour may be dictated by what aspect they happen to be focusing on at any one particular time.

Expectation and perception

Expectation works in a similar way to motivation. Myers and Myers (1992) state that people are more likely to pay attention to aspects of their environment that they expect than to those they do not expect. For this reason therefore we may not always perceive things as they really are.

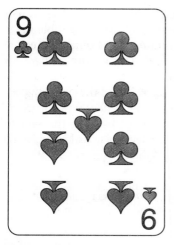

Figure 5.8(a)
Nine of Clubs or nine of Spades depending on where you are looking

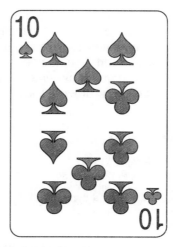

Figure 5.8(b)
Ten of Spades or ten of Clubs depending on where you are looking

Time

Perception is influenced by time in that the longer we are exposed to something the more we will perceive that thing. There is also another side to the effect of long exposure to a particular stimulus. The longer we are exposed to something, the more likely it is to blend into the background. An example would be the constant playing of music, sometimes we hardly notice it is there. Similarly if you have experienced entering a room that has a strange smell, you only notice the smell for a few minutes or so, longer exposure tends to make your olfactory sense (in this particular case) become accustomed to that strange smell.

The scoring for Exercise 26 can be worked out in the following way. Questions 1, 2, 3, 4, 9, 12, 14, 17, 20, 21, 22, and 23 are keyed in as False to indicate a tendency for high self-monitoring. Similarly items 5, 6, 7, 8, 10, 11, 13, 15, 16, 18, 19, 24, and 25 are keyed in as True to indicate high self-monitoring. For example if you have answered 'false' to question 1, 'I find it difficult to copy the behaviour of other people' (a false statement), your tendency is towards high self-monitoring. Similarly if you have answered 'true' for question 8, 'I would probably make a good actor,' this would suggest your tendency towards high self-monitoring.

Perception and self-awareness

One could argue that an awareness of one's own perception holds the key to the way one interacts with others. Behaviour is inextricably linked with perception and this is clearly indicated in O'Connor and Seymour's (1990) model of communication. For example through awareness of my own perception, I will come to realise that what I see depends on my perspective of the object. Everything depends on my internal frame of reference. If I am depressed, I will see life as worthless and if I am happy, I will see life as exciting. Similarly if I can only see your negative side, then I will see you as negative. An awareness of my internal frame of reference will enable me to have an undiluted view of others. In order to understand others, I need to recognise and accept my own internal responses. This in turn will enable me to recognise and accept the internal responses of others. Recognising and accepting others for who they are is one of the foci of the next chapter.

References

Bandura, A. (1974). 'Behaviour Theory and the model of man.' *American Psychologist*, **29**, 859–869.

Baron, R.A. and Byrne, D. (1991). *Social Psychology. Understanding Human Interaction.* Boston, London, Toronto, Sydney, Tokyo, Singapore: Allyn and Bacon.

Chance, P. (1989). 'Seeing is believing. Even though what you see is not necessarily what you get.' *Psychology Today*, **23**, 26.

Duck, S. (1997). *Handbook of Personal Relationship.* New York: Wiley.

Hamachek, D. (1992). *Encounters with Self.* London: Harcourt Brace Jovanovich College Publishers.

Hastorft, H.A., Schneider, D.J. and Ppolefka, J. (1970). *Person Perception.* Reading, MA: Addison-Wesley.

Heider, F. (1958). *The Psychology of Interpersonal Relations.* New York: John Wiley and Sons, Inc. London: Chapman and Hall.

Icheiser, G. (1949). 'Misunderstandings in human relations.' *American Journal of Sociology*, **55**, 2, Part 2.

Leeper, R. (1935). 'The role of motivation in learning. A study of the phenomenon of differential motivation control of the utilisation of habits.' *Journal of Genetic Psychology*, **46**, 3–40.

Myers, G.E. and Myers, M.T. (1992). *The Dynamics of Human Communication: A Laboratory Approach.* London: McGraw-Hill.

O'Connor, J. and Seymour, J. (1990). *Introducing Neurolinguistic Programming. Psychological Skills for Understanding and Influencing People.* London: Aquarian.

Piaget, J. (1952). *The Origins of Intelligence in Children.* New York: International Universities Press.

Snyder, M. (1974). 'Self monitoring of expressive behaviour.' *Journal of Personality and Social Psychology*, **30**, 526–537.

Snyder, M. (1987). *Public Appearances Private Realities: The Psychology of Self-Monitoring.* New York: W.H. Freeman and Company.

Snyder, M., Gangestad, S. and Simpson, J.A. (1983). 'Choosing friends as activity partners:- The role of self monitoring.' *Journal of Personality and Social Psychology*, **45**, 1061–1072.

A humanistic point of view

6

Objectives

After reading this chapter you should be able to:

1   Discuss the eclectical nature of humanistic perspective
2   Explain some of the existential philosophical principles which underpin the humanistic perspective
3   Discuss Maslow's (1954) theory of motivation
4   Explain the notion of individual as an 'integrated whole'
5   Discuss some of the characteristics of a self-actualiser
6   Discuss Rogers' (1951) self theory
7   Understand the notion of phenomenology
8   Explain self-concept and organismic valuing process
9   Differentiate between positive regards, positive self regard, condition of worth, conditional and unconditional positive regards, congruence and incongruence

Eclectic approach

Both Abraham Maslow and Carl Rogers brought a new dimension to the concept of caring. This is seen particularly in counselling but perhaps more so in nursing. These psychologists came from the school of thought which is commonly known as Humanistic. Maslow is credited with being the founder of humanistic psychology (Hjelle and Ziegler, 1992). Humanistic perspective can be seen as, not just one single organised theory, it is instead based on numerous principles, some of which are from psychoanalytical and behavioural thoughts. In this sense it can be described as an eclectic perspective. Maslow called it a third force psychology because prior to emergence of humanism, the two predominant forces were psychoanalytic and behavioural.

Third force psychology

Existential philosophy

Some of the underpinning principles of humanistic psychology rest within what is described as existential philosophy. An existentialist approach focuses on the person's concrete and specific consciousness of existing at a particular time in space. The implication is that people are consciously aware of their own existence and eventual death. People are aware that they exist as they live and they cease to exist when they die. The main emphasis of who we are and what we become is focused around the idea that we alone are responsible for who or what we become. Existentialists discard the nature versus nurture debate and believe that people are the makers of their own destiny.

Existential principles indicate that each and every one individual is

- a unique individual
- aware of his/her own experience
- the creator and controller of his/her own destiny
- completely free to make his/her choices
- responsible for his/her own existence

Life is what we make of it

Existentialists believe that life is what an individual makes of it. The key issue however is that of genuineness and honesty. The big question is whether people can be honest and genuine in the way they live their lives. The concept of existentialism was very appealing to the humanists and in their quest for a new approach they adopted many of its sentiments. Humanists further believe that

Principles of humanistic philosophy

- each individual is the chief determinant of his or her behaviour and experience
- humans are conscious agents, experiencing, deciding and freely choosing their own actions
- becoming or self-actualising, which basically means a person is never static, he or she is always in the process of becoming something different
- it is the individual's responsibility as a free agent to realise as many of his or her potentialities as possible
- people who refuse to become, refuse to grow. They have denied themselves the full possibilities of human existence
- human consciousness, subjective feelings, moods and personal experiences are crucial because they all relate to one's existence in the world of other people

Maslow (1908–1970) and his theory of motivation

The starting point of this discussion is with the works of Maslow. Maslow believed that

1 Each individual has an 'inner nature which is in part unique to ourselves and in part species-wide' (Maslow, 1968, p.3).
2 People are not born evil, but if they are destructive, sadistic and cruel, it is because their intrinsic needs, their emotions and capacities are frustrated.
3 People should be encouraged to express their inner nature, which is basically good, and if they are guided they would grow healthily.

4   People's inner nature is weak, delicate and can be easily overcome
by habit and cultural pressure.

Maslow believed that an individual is an integrated and organised   ***The individual is an***
whole and as such when we study people, we have to look at them in the   ***integrated whole***
same light. If we chose to look at the individual as separate bits and pieces,
all we will get is a snapshot of one small piece of a jigsaw, the complete
picture will elude us. 'In good theory there is no such entity as a need of
the stomach or mouth, or a genital need. There is only a need of the individual. It is John Smith who wants food, not John Smith's stomach'
(Maslow, 1954, p.63). Ask yourself the following questions.

Who wants food, you or your stomach?
Who wants sex, you or your genitals?
Who wants to see the latest blockbuster movie, you or your eyes?
Who wants to listen to nice music, you or your ears?

The most obvious answer is 'you' and not the different parts of your body.
Although simplistic in nature, these questions stress the point that if one
is to make sense of human behaviour then one needs to look at people in
a holistic way.

Motivation can be described as the energising force of behaviour.   ***Theory of motivation***
Maslow argued that people's behaviour can be understood by their ten-
dency to seek personal goal which makes life rewarding and meaningful.
From this perspective one could say that Maslow's basic tenet was that the
driving force of behaviour is motivation. 'Man is a wanting animal and
rarely reaches a state of complete satisfaction except for a short time. As
one desire is satisfied, another pops up to take its place. When this is satisfied still another comes into the foreground, etc. It is a characteristic of
the human being throughout his whole life that he is practically always
desiring something' (Maslow, 1954, p.69).

Figure 6.1
*A diagrammatical representation of
Maslow's Hierarchy of Needs*

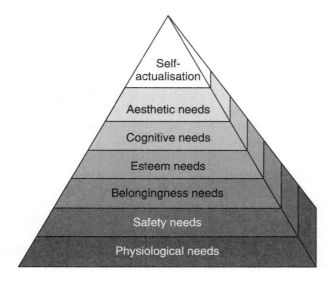

Maslow suggested that all human needs are instinctoid, what he meant by this is that one is born with them. These needs are arranged in an ascending hierarchical order based on the priority of satisfaction. These basic needs are identified as

1   Physiological needs
2   Safety needs
3   Belongingness and love needs
4   Esteem needs
5   The desire to know and to understand needs (cognitive needs)
6   Aesthetic needs
7   Self-actualisation needs

Physiological needs

Maslow stated that the physiological needs are usually taken as the starting point for motivation theory. These needs include food, water, air, and sex. The scenario is that if people are hungry as well as lacking in safety, love and esteem, their behaviour will most likely be driven by the hunger rather than by any of the other drives. Satisfying their hunger becomes the utmost priority. 'For the man who is extremely, and dangerously hungry, no other interests exist but food. He dreams of food, he remembers food, he thinks of food, and he emotes only about food, he perceives only food and he wants only food' (Maslow, 1954, p.82). As soon as the individual's basic desire for food is satisfied, then other needs classed as higher order needs will emerge.

Safety needs

Only when people's tummies are full, will they start to look for safety and security. This therefore becomes the driving force of their future behaviour. Maslow stated that a child's need for safety is seen in his preference for a routine with some element of sameness. People would not like their routine to be disrupted. They seem to want a predictable and orderly world. For example injustice, unfairness, and lack of consistency in the parents' behaviour would make a child feel insecure and anxious. Some of the things which threaten security are quarrelling, physical assault, separation, divorce or death within the family. In an adult the need for safety and security can be seen in the need for a permanent job, owning one's own house, and establishing financial security. Satisfaction of the safety and security needs triggers off the need for belongingness and love.

Belongingness and love needs

Maslow argued that when both the physiological and safety needs have been satisfied, the individual can feel free to pursue love, affection and belongingness. The person will miss the company of friends, or a sweetheart, or a wife, or children. People will develop a hunger for an affectionate relationship within their group. Wanting to love and be loved becomes a key feature at this stage in the hierarchy of needs. Having said that, love is not seen as synonymous with sex. Sex, Maslow argued can be taken as a purely physiological need.

The esteem needs

People have a need for a positive evaluation of themselves. They need self-respect, self-esteem , respect and esteem from others. If these needs are satisfied, people will feel confident, with a sense of worth, they will come to believe that they stand for something and that they have a sense of purpose in life. However, if these needs are thwarted, people will be left with feelings of inferiority, and helplessness. Parental influences are seen as extremely important in instilling positive self-esteem in children. If a child is brought with the feeling of worthiness and love, this child will grow up to feel good about himself or herself. Similarly if a child is deprived of a sense of worth and love, he or she will grow up feeling insecure and negative about himself or herself. Maslow stated that the most healthy self-esteem is based on deserved respect from others and not on fame and celebrity. This suggests an element of dynamism between self and others, respect from others has to be worked for.

The need for self-actualisation

If all the needs that have already been discussed are satisfied, there will still emerge another need, which is related to what this individual is fit for. For example musicians must express themselves in their music, artists must express themselves in their painting, and poets must express themselves in their writing. And only then will they be at peace with themselves. This ultimate expression, that is to become who an individual is capable of becoming, is what Maslow called self-actualisation. Maslow said that the word self-actualisation refers to a person's desire for self-fulfilment, and this suggests becoming what one is able to become. This can be described as follows, if a car's top speed is 100 m.p.h., then self-actualisation for the car will be reached if it attains this maximum speed. Maslow (1970), phrased this as the desire to become more and more what one is, to become. Self-actualisation is very much a personal phenomenon and people have their own actualisation. Completion of this book may do it for me, whereas for you, it may be obtaining your diploma, your degree or your PhD.

The characteristics of a self-actualiser are said to include

Portrait of a self-actualiser

- being able to perceive reality efficiently and being comfortable with it
- being much more able to accept self and others
- behaving spontaneously
- tendency to problem focus rather than self-centred
- needing privacy and solitude
- self reliant for own growth and development
- tendency to engage in deeper and more satisfying interpersonal relationships with a few rather than many people

- ability to discriminate between means and ends
- possessing an air of creativity

Peak experiences

Hjelle and Ziegler (1992) describe Maslow's concept of peak experience as the periods when people feel great ecstasy. In his attempt to discover the meaning of peak experiences, Maslow (1971, pp.174–175) asked people such questions as

- What was the most ecstatic moment of your life?
- Have you experienced transcendent ecstasy?
- What was the single most joyous, happiest, most blissful moment of your whole life?
- How did you feel different about yourself at that time?
- How did the world look different?
- What did you feel like?
- What were your impulses?
- How did you change, if you did?

Maslow concluded from the way people answered these questions, that there exist such a concept and in fact almost everyone has peak experiences of ecstasies. From Maslow's own perspective, two of the easiest ways of getting peak experiences are through music and through sex. It is not difficult to understand that sex can in fact lead to the most blissful experience in one's life, especially during orgasm. While some people may have their rapturous experience listening to Chopin, Mozart, Vivaldi, Bon Jovi, Boy Zone, or even The Spice Girls, I have my blissful moments listening to Celine Dion, I have to add however not to the point of orgasm.

The need to know and to understand

Maslow believed that everyone has a need to know and understand what goes on around him or her. This would include the search for knowledge, the discovery of new world, the exploration of a mysterious land, and so on. Maslow (1954) stated that studying psychologically healthy people reveals a defining characteristic of being attracted to mysteries and to the unknown. There is an element within every individual that wants to know what is in a black box. Watching a child taking a toy apart is not an unusual occurrence and certainly from Maslow's point of view monkeys will pick things apart, will poke their fingers into holes, will explore every unknown situation. From a human perspective, if one sees a different coloured cloud in the sky, one wants to know why; if one hears a loud noise, one wants to know the source. Perhaps the need to know does not carry similar intensity as the other basic needs; having said that, it does contribute to the other needs in the sense that the people need to know where their food will come from, where safety lies, who thinks highly or lowly of them. Maslow said that insight is usually a bright and happy emotional state in anyone's life.

The aesthetic needs

The aesthetic needs, of all the other needs, are rather difficult to conceptualise, but the nearest one can get to it is to imagine how pleasant things are appreciated, and how ugly things make the individual feel uncomfortable. Perhaps the best explanation of the aesthetic needs rest in Maslow's (1954, p.97) words, 'what, for instance, does it mean when a man feels a strong conscious impulse to straighten the crookedly hung picture on the wall?' This suggests that the individual has a need to seek for beauty and pleasant things. Which would you prefer to watch, a fashion show or a television scene where there are human miseries through wars or droughts? If I am not mistaken, it is most likely you will choose the fashion show because it is a more pleasant experience.

Although the needs that Maslow identified have been placed in an hierarchical order based on the urgency of their satisfaction, that is, if I am both starving and unprotected, the chances are that I will be driven by my hunger to search for food and only when my hunger is wholly or partly satisfied, will I look for a place to stay. Maslow pointed out that this may not be the same in every case and here are some exceptions.

Some people may have a different hierarchy of needs

- For some people self-esteem may be more important than love and belongingness.
- Others may see creativity as taking precedence over most of the other basic needs.
- In Maslow's words, a person who is chronically unemployed, may continue to be satisfied for the rest of his life if only he can get enough food.
- Some people may not know what love is, for example, if they have never had love, they would not know what love was and thus love would not feature in their hierarchy of needs.
- Similarly if one never knows what starvation feels like and food has always been in abundance one may not come to realise the importance of this particular need, so one may perceive other higher needs as more important.
- Maslow claimed that people will want the more basic of the two needs when deprived of both, but he did not imply that people will act on their desires. This can be conceived of as 'wanting something is one thing but going for it a completely different thing altogether'.
- Finally people's sense of morals and values may well dictate the hierarchy of their basic needs, like political activists, suicide bombers and martyrs.

In order to understand the concept of motivation based on an hierarchy of needs, there are certain factors which Maslow stressed upon and these include

- Satisfaction of needs does not imply that these needs have to be satisfied fully, they could be satisfied partially, depending on the individual.
- These needs are taken in general to be unconscious in nature, one has to recognise however that some of these needs may become conscious.

- Although there may be some cultural specificity, that is, some cultures may have different hierarchical priorities, nevertheless there exist some elements of commonness.
- Most behaviours are multimotivated. This means that one is not motivated by just one single drive or factor.
- One's behaviour is not necessarily determined by basic needs, some may be determined by the situation one finds oneself in. Some behaviour is highly motivated whilst other behaviour may be weakly motivated and still other behaviour may not be motivated at all.

Deficiency and growth motivation

Deficiency motives

Maslow (1968) identified two categories of motives and these are deficiency and growth. The characteristics of deficiency motives (D Types Motives) are

- if a basic need is missing, one would become ill
- the presence of this need would prevent illness
- the restoration of such a need will cure the illness
- under certain situations which suggest a certain element of free choice, the basic need is preferred by the deprived person over other satisfactions
- the basic needs are found to be inactive or functionally absent in the healthy person

Growth motives

The growth motives, also called Metaneeds or B-Motives, focus on enriching and expanding one's experience of living. In this sense it could be said that the growth motives are secondary to the deficiency motives.

Carl Rogers (1902–1987) and the self theory

Maslow and Rogers like so many of the humanists, had a lot in common as far as their beliefs in human nature were concerned. Rogers' emphasis however, was mainly on the phenomenological point of view. The word phenomenology means the study of an individual's subjective experience. This experience is believed to be unique to that person.

A phenomenological perspective

Rogers' (1951) theory of personality and behaviour is based on 19 propositions, a summary of these is offered here. Some of Rogers' key concepts will be integrated into the discussion.

People exist in a continually changing world of experience

Rogers' concept of 'Phenomenal Field', can be roughly translated to mean the sum total of the person's experience and this experience encompasses both what is conscious and what is unconscious. Conscious and unconscious are likened to figure and ground respectively, with conscious in the foreground and unconscious residing in the background. Only a small portion of this experience is conscious, but the rest can emerge from the unconscious depending on the needs of the person. Rogers (1951, p.483) stated, 'Most of the individual's experiences constitute the ground of the perceptual field, but they can easily become figure, while other experiences slip back into ground.' Have a look at Figures 6.2 and 6.3, this may simplify Rogers' point further. Rogers said that the only person who can know how the experience was perceived is that particular individual. It would also be true to say that the experiencer is better placed than any other individual to know of that experience. The organism reacts to the field as it is experienced and perceived. This perceptual field is, for the individual, 'reality'. The basic sentiment from this statement is that both 'you and I see what we see and behave accordingly'. The emphasis here is that reality is an individual thing. Your reality is not my reality. This concept becomes more meaningful when one's reality is compared with that of a person suffering from hallucinations. It is easy to say that this particular person is living in a different world with a different reality.

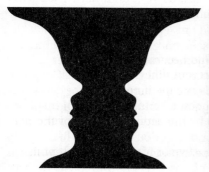

Figure 6.2
Shows a black vase

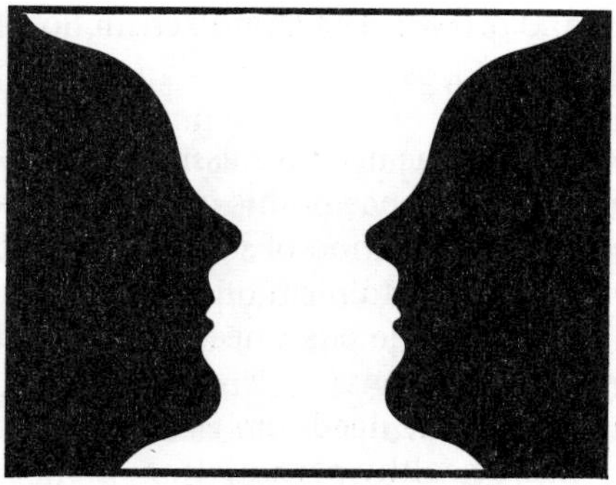

Figure 6.3
Shows the silhouettes of two human faces

The black vase in Figure 6.2 is more prominent than the two white facial silhouettes. Similarly in Figure 6.3, the two human silhouettes facing each other are more prominent than the white vase. Whatever you see when you look at either Figure 6.2 or 6.3, this suggests that you are consciously aware of that image at that particular time. Whether you see a black vase or a couple of black human silhouettes depends on your awareness in time.

This falls into the concept of holism, one reacts to any situation as a whole organism rather than with specific parts of one's body, for example if a person's little toe hurts, the whole of that person suffers, not just his or her little toe.

The organism reacts as a whole to this phenomenal field

Rogers' self-actualisation concept is similar to that of Maslow and it suggests that one's goal in life is to seek to move forward and develop one's existence to its fullest. Rogers (1951, p.488) stated, 'We are speaking of the tendency of the organism to move in the direction of maturation, as maturation is defined for each species.' Given a choice, one would prefer to be healthy rather than sick, self dependent rather than depending on others, and to achieve that which one is capable of achieving.

People tend to strive for self-actualisation

Rogers argued that behaviour is a goal-directed attempt on behalf of the organism to satisfy its needs as is perceived and experienced. This can be interpreted as, I perceive and experience my needs and my behaviour

Behaviour is directed towards the needs of the person

therefore is directed towards satisfying those needs. Rogers suggested here that emotion of whichever type, plays a role in any goal-directed behaviour. People do things and the importance these things have in their lives, will dictate their emotional arousal.

The best way to understand people is from their point of view

Rogers stressed the sentiment that if one wants to understand a person's behaviour, then one has to look at it from the person's perspective. If we do not, then all we will see is our perspective of that particular person's behaviour and sadly, that will not mean much. A small cut on an individual's finger might be a big problem for him or her, whereas this may seem trivial to someone else. Rogers' focus was individuals and their interactions with the environment as they perceive it to exist.

Unitary whole

Self-concept

Rogers argued that when infants are born, at first they are not able to differentiate between themselves and the environment. Babies perceive all their experiences as unitary wholes and do not have the capacity to work out what is 'me' and what is 'not me'. Self as such does not exist at that time. As they gradually develop and interact with the environment, they develop ideas as to what is 'me,' 'I,' and 'myself'. This could be seen as the initial stage of the development of the self-concept. Rogers stressed that his usage of the term 'self' differs from 'organism' in that the former is more to do with the 'awareness of being'. Rogers used the terms self, self-concept, and self structure interchangeably. Self-concept therefore can be defined as 'the organised, consistent conceptual gestalt composed of the perceptions of the characteristics of the "I" or "me" and the perceptions of the relationships of the "I" or "me" to others and to various aspects of life, together with the values attached to these perceptions. It is a gestalt which is available to awareness though not necessarily in awareness' (Rogers, 1959, p.200).

Self-image

The self-concept is a reflection of what people perceive themselves to be. This includes those characteristics that they perceive as part of themselves like their physical attributes such as height, hair colour and the way one dresses. Self-image can also mean the roles one occupies in society, for example husband, father, son, daughter, mother, student, lecturer and so on.

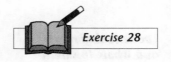

Exercise 28

Make a list of your (a) physical attributes and (b) roles that you have in society. Whatever you come up with, this will be your self-image. If for example you describe yourself with derogatory adjectives, one would say that you hold a negative self-image. Similarly if you are complimentary about your attributes, you will be seen as having a positive self-image.

Self-esteem

A further dimension of self-concept is self-esteem. This is described as the value or worth which one imposes on oneself. The word esteem may suggest a high regard, in this context it is seen to have both a positive and a negative valence or pole. If for example I think positively of myself, I would be described as having high self-esteem. Similarly if I think of myself in a negative way, then I would be perceived to have low self-esteem. Both self-image and self-esteem have direct influences on one's behaviour. Positive self-image and high self-esteem lead to confident and assertive behaviour. Similarly negative self-image and low self-esteem lead to unassertive behaviour or behaviour which shows a lack of confidence.

According to Rogers, infants interact with the environment and formulate impressions of themselves and the environment. Through this dynamism they become aware of which experiences are pleasant and which are not pleasant. They are then able to work out that the pleasant experiences enhance, where as the unpleasant experiences hinder, their growth and development. Children develop ongoing processes during which they make value judgements based on the evidence from their own senses. Rogers referred to this phenomenon as organismic valuing process. 'There soon enters into this picture the evaluation of self by others. "You're a good child," "You're a naughty boy." These and similar evaluations of himself and of his behaviour by his parents and others come to form a large and significant part of the infant's perceptual field' (Rogers, 1951, p.499).

Organismic valuing process

Although those behaviours which children exhibit are satisfying to them, they may not necessarily be satisfying to their parents. Rogers stated that children pick up cues about which behaviour receives approval and which does not. Those behaviours which stimulate parental disapproval lead them to conclude that they are bad. If their behaviour is seen as bad, therefore they cannot be loveable.

Introjection

Children are in conflict, because although parents do not approve, these behaviours are nevertheless satisfying in themselves. Rogers said that children deal with this conflict in one of two ways. They may deny that the behaviour was satisfying or they may distort the symbolisation of the parents' experience. What this means is that children behave as though these were their own experiences and that the behaviours were in fact unsatisfactory. So instead of 'My parents see this behaviour as unsatisfactory (as it should really be), it becomes, 'I see this behaviour as unsatisfactory'. This is what Rogers called introjection. The individual takes on board the feelings or thoughts of his or her parents and behaves as if they are his or hers. This is not dissimilar to Berne's concept of racket feeling (see Chapter 7).

Development of self-concept

According to Rogers, there are certain factors which contribute to a positive self-concept. These include the universal need for positive regard. Everyone has a desire to be loved and accepted by significant others. Rogers believed that people will do almost anything to gain positive regard and will even be prepared to put on hold their organismic valuing systems. They also have a need for positive self-regard, this basically suggests a need to love and to accept themselves.

Positive regard and positive self-regard

We know that the need for positive regard is such that we are prepared to go to any lengths to ensure that we get it. We also pick up cues from significant others that certain behaviours will lead to receiving positive regard and other behaviours will not. When positive regard is contingent on good behaviour, then this is called condition of worth. When positive regard is dependent on conditions of worth, this is called conditional positive regards. From Rogers perspective, both conditions of worth and con-

Conditions of worth

Conditional positive regards

Unconditional positive regard

ditional positive regard are detrimental to growth and development. When positive regard is given irrespective of someone's worth, this is called unconditional positive regard. Unconditional positive regard is a prerequisite skill for health care professionals, whatever one's discipline happens to be.

Rogers argued that as people experience life, their experiences are structured in one of three ways, and these are

- symbolised, perceived, and organised into some relationship to the self
- ignored because there is no perceived relationship to self structure
- denied symbolisation or given a distorted symbolisation because the experience is inconsistent with the structure of self

Roughly translated this could be taken to mean

- if the experience means nothing to me I do not see it and it is insignificant
- if I perceive myself as not fitting in the particular context, then I do not engage
- if I have a low opinion of myself, and people give me compliment, I do not believe them because it is not consistent with the way I feel

One behaves therefore in ways which are consistent with how one sees oneself, for example if I see myself as a confident person, I will behave in a confident manner, similarly if I perceive myself as weak then my behaviour will reflect that perception. Having said that, I may do something (as a result of a pressing urge), which is not in keeping with my self-concept, and then my rationale for such a behaviour could be 'I don't know what came over me'.

Congruence and incongruence

Rogers believed that psychological maladjustment exists when the organism denies his or her experiences. These experiences are then not symbolised in one's self structure and this leads to a situation of potential psychological tension. This is as if my feeling is in the ground (in a figure and ground context) and I dare not let it become the figure because this does not fit in with my self-concept. I may feel a certain dislike towards my students, but because I perceive myself as a good teacher, I cannot tell them that I dislike them. This dynamism, if experienced, will generate tension which could eventually hinder growth and development. The word incongruence is appropriate here and this suggests that there is a lack of harmony and hence a discrepancy exists between what the person experiences and his or her self-concept. The situation however is not altogether hopeless, because through assimilation of new information, I could come to grips with the idea that sometimes 'If this is the way I feel then this is the way I feel'. I basically restructure my thinking and review my self-concept so that I am able to accommodate this new way of looking at myself and I no longer feel any tension when my behaviour is congruent with my feelings. A state of congruence between how one feels and how one behaves is the recipe for good interpersonal relationships. The words congruence, transparency and genuineness would seem to carry similar sentiments.

Humanism and caring

Rogers would argue that if helpers can accept themselves as they truly are, and feel what they truly experience, then they will be more able to accept others as separate individuals. The sentiment here seems to suggest that self-awareness and self-acceptance are the avenues to accepting others. As individuals perceive and come to accept their true self-concept, they would be able to do what they think they should do rather than what they think others want them to do, they would be able to function according to their organismic valuing processes. Relying on one's organismic valuing process will make one a fully functioning person. This means that individuals are able to experience their feelings, and as such will not be afraid of any of them. Emotions and feeling are the focus of the next chapter.

References

Hjelle, L.A. and Ziegler, D.J. (1992). *Personality Theories. Basic Assumptions, Research, and Applications.* New York: McGraw-Hill International Editions.

Maslow, A.H. (1954). *Motivation and Personality.* New York: Harper and Row.

Maslow, A.H. (1968). *Towards a Psychology of Being.* New York: Van Nostrand.

Maslow, A.H. (1970). *Motivation and Personality.* New York: Harper and Row.

Maslow, A.H. (1971). *The Farther Reaches of Human Nature.* New York: Viking Press.

Rogers, C.R. (1951). *Client Centred Therapy.* London: Constable.

Rogers, C.R. (1959). 'A Theory of therapy, personality and interpersonal relationships, as developed in the client-centred framework.' In: Koch, S. (Ed.) *Psychology: A Study of a Science,* Vol. 3, New York: McGraw-Hill, pp. 184–256.

Rogers, C.R. (1961). *On Becoming A Person: A Therapist's View of Psychotherapy.* London: Constable.

Emotion and behaviour 7

Objectives

After reading this chapter you should be able to:

1   Discuss the relevance of emotion to communication
2   Explain some of the characteristics of emotion
3   Differentiate between appropriate and inappropriate emotion
4   Explain the social function of emotion
5   Describe the dynamics of some emotions
6   Recognise anger as a normal appropriate emotion
7   Discuss some of the psychological theories of anger
8   Explain some of the functions of anger
9   Understand the relationship between emotion and care delivery

Emotion: the very essence of being

What is a person without emotion? A person without emotion can be likened to a body without a heart. A world without emotion would be a world full of androids, with expressionless and meaningless faces. Emotions have always been of central concern to everyone and they are involved in practically everything that one does. Emotion allows an individual to be able to appreciate and recognise love, pain and grief, among the numerous other things. No study or literature on communication would be complete without at least mentioning the word emotion. Certainly emotion can be described as the very essence of being. From an evolutionary approach, emotion is described as the very essence of all animal communication and its expression can be seen through the various form of verbal, non-verbal and paralanguage. Referring to Buck's theory Plutchik (1994, p.95) explains, 'when emotions occur, an emotional state is encoded in the central nervous system and expressed or sent by means of facial expressions, sounds, or gestures. The receiver attends to these signals, decodes them, and uses the information received in accord with his or her own motivational or emotional state.'

The problem which emotion has always posed to theorists is that of definition. Everyone knows what emotion is by experiencing it, but how does one explain what one means by the term. It is very difficult indeed to define this construct. Harre (1986) says that there are in fact about 400 words for emotion in English. What is known about emotion is that it has at least three characteristics and these are physiological, expressive and experiential.

Physiological aspect

The physiological aspect of emotion is believed to have its roots in the limbic system of the brain. For example arousal of particular parts of the limbic system leads to changes in heart rate, sweating and blood pressure. According to Delgado (1971) electrical stimulation of the brain (ESB) resulted in two types of emotional response. For example when the part of the brain which is called the anterior hypothalamus is stimulated in cats, this produces what is described as a false rage (pseudorage). Pseudorage is basically a vocal display of aggressive behaviour (hissing and growling) which is not directed at other cats even when the stimulated animal is being attacked. Stimulation of the cat's lateral hypothalamus on the other hand produced true aggressive display to ward off the threatening danger. Delgado (1971) cited in Izard (1977, p.114) said that stimulation of the right amygdala (part of the limbic system) 'produced "a fit of rage" in a psychiatric patient who was playing a guitar and singing when she was stimulated by remote control radio signal'.

Expressive aspect

The expressive aspect of emotion is related to facial expression, vocal cues, body movements and facial expression (see Figure 7.1).

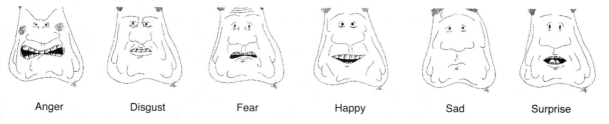

| Anger | Disgust | Fear | Happy | Sad | Surprise |

Figure 7.1
The different faces of emotion

Experiential aspect

The experiential aspect of emotion is believed to be crucial to daily functioning in that it may be responsible for motivating action.

According to Plutchik and Kellerman (1980), there are eight primary emotions and these are

* acceptance
* disgust

- anticipation/expectation
- anger
- fear
- joy
- sadness and
- surprise

Mixed emotion

Combinations of these emotions lead to secondary emotions and these include

- aggressiveness (anger + anticipation)
- awe (fear + surprise)
- contempt (anger + disgust)
- disappointment (sadness + surprise)
- love (acceptance + joy)
- optimism (anticipation + joy)
- remorse (sadness + disgust)
- submission (acceptance + fear)

Mixed emotion is perhaps a difficult concept to follow. In reality however, the way people behave clearly suggests elements of mixed emotions. Consider the following scenario.

My son informs me that he is going out and should be back in 2 hours. Two hours pass by, and I keep thinking he will be home soon. Another 2 hours and still no sign of him. My anger level has gradually risen during that time and at the back of my mind there is this niggling doubt that something may have happened to him. Then all of a sudden the door opens and my son appears. I feel a sense of relief and it is really good to know he is home safe. No sooner said, I then feel the urge to express my anger by saying, 'couldn't you have called?' 'I have been worried sick wondering where you are,' and 'by the way if you want any food, you'll just have to make it yourself'.

Mixed emotions are evident in the above scenario and a closer look reveals at least three emotions at play and these are anger, anticipation and relief. I was angry because my son did not keep his promise of returning at the stated time. My anticipation was that something untoward may have happened to him. I felt a sense of relief to see him safe.

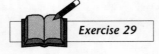

Exercise 29

Reflect on some of the times when you have experienced mixed emotions. Explore the different emotions at play and share these with someone, a colleague or your best friend.

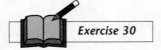

Exercise 30

Have you always expressed your true feelings? Reflect and recall any situations when you have not expressed your true feelings. Try and establish the reason, if any, as to why you did not express your true feelings.

The rationale for Exercise 30 is that some would argue that there may have been times when people do not express how they truly feel. This is especially so if they know that the felt emotion does nothing towards expressing their true feelings. Another reason for not expressing one's true feelings is that one may not know any better. Basically the person could have learned this behaviour from parents or significant others. Say for example I condemn the expression of sadness or grief and every time any member of my family makes an attempt to express sadness as they feel it, I demonstrate my disapproval by being angry. As this continues, my children would grow up to believe that the emotion of sadness should not be expressed but anger through aggressive behaviour is acceptable. What may happen is that instead of showing grief my children may show anger even if anger is not the appropriate emotion. They would have learned to put their true feelings on hold and take on a substitute feeling. This is called a racket feeling and the reason for this is that the feeling displayed is not a true representation of the felt emotion. It needs to be stressed here that the acquisition of racket feelings can be an unconscious phenomenon.

Racket feeling

. . . He knows if you've been bad or good,
so be good for goodness sake.

Oh, You'd better watch out,
You'd better not cry.
You'd better not pout,
I'm telling you why,

'Cos, Santa Claus is coming to town,
Santa Claus is coming to town,
Santa Claus is coming to town.

H. Gillespie and J. Coots (1970) 'Santa Claus is Coming to Town'

The above lyrics from a Christmas song entitled, 'Santa Claus is Coming to Town,' by the Jackson 5 seems to suggest that if the child is not good, Santa will not like it. The 'not good' concept is linked with crying. If the child cries, then this is bad. Although innocent in its intention, nevertheless it does give young children the message that they are bad if they cry and that crying does not carry a reward. From this aspect, parents are not the only culprits in inducing racket feelings in children. In fact almost any one can, and does so.

Be good, don't cry

So the big question is, 'did you at any time display any racket feeling?' Perhaps some of the following statements will help to jog your memory.

- Grin and bare it
- Don't let them know how you feel
- Don't cry you'll look silly
- What will the neighbours say if they hear you shouting?
- Don't be upset

- Pretend it does not hurt
- If you are given a present you dislike, say, 'thank you, that's what I have always wanted'

Appropriate and inappropriate emotion

Racket feelings are good examples of the so-called inappropriate emotions. Armon-Jones defines an inappropriate emotion as 'one which is not warranted by the evoking object or situation' (Harre, 1986, p.67). By contrast an appropriate emotion is one whose arousal is congruent with the evoking object or situation. For example I am fearful of crocodiles because they are dangerous and laughing in the face of a crocodile would be inappropriate. Similarly if you are to tell me that I have won the lottery, the appropriate emotion would be one of joy, so it would be natural for me to be happy. Having said that, there are many people who cry with joy and although this could be seen as inappropriate, one argument would be that the true emotional expression is one of joy to the happy event. If on the other hand you are to give me some bad news and instead of expressing sadness or sorrow, I burst into laughter, it is most likely that I would be said to be suffering from incongruity of affect.

The social functions of emotion

Does emotion have a function other than letting others know how one is feeling? Armon-Jones (1986) states that according to constructionism, emotion contributes to the preservation of the moral rules of society. For example if I should feel guilty regarding a deed which I have committed, from a constructionistic perspective I would not repeat the same deed again because of the way it makes me feel afterwards (I am merely presenting a non-evaluative perspective regarding the functions of emotion and as such I shall not engage in arguing the point). Parents would on numerous occasions use emotion as a means of instilling moral values into their children with such statements like, 'You should be ashamed of yourself' and 'You ought to feel bad for the way you behaved'. From this particular point of view one could say that emotion serves a social function.

The dynamics of emotions

Plutchik (1994) identifies nine derivatives for each of the emotions, here however only four of them are considered in relation to the felt emotion. These derivatives are:

1 The event
2 Perception of the event
3 Felt emotion
4 Behavioural response

Event

The event underpins the felt emotion, for example what in the environment is responsible for the arousal of any particular emotion. As Plutchik (1984) says, 'all emotions are triggered by events that have an important

Table 7.1
Emotions and some of their derivatives. Adapted from Plutchik (1994)

Stimulus event	Perception of event	Felt emotion	Behavioural response
Threat	Danger	Fear	Escape
Obstacle	Enemy	Anger	Attack
Potential mate	Possess	Joy	Mate
Loss (loved one)	Abandonment	Sadness	Cry
Member of one's group	Friend	Acceptance	Groom
Unpalatable object	Poison	Disgust	Vomit
New territory	What's out there?	Expectation	Map
Unexpected object	What is it?	Surprise	Stop

significance for the organism' (Scherer and Ekman, 1984, p.212). Table 7.1 shows examples of some of the events.

Perception of the event is very much an individual phenomenon which is based on one's own frame of reference.   ***Perception of the event***

Felt emotion is the actual arousal which in most cases is the expressive aspect.   ***Felt emotion***

Behavioural response is the actual act which follows the arousal and this can be anything from running away to an aggressive display.   ***Behavioural response***

Anger

Anger is something which every individual has experienced at one time or another. It is an emotion and all emotions can be seen as states of arousal which are caused by the situation which people find themselves in, for example fear is arousal plus the thoughts of escape, disgust is arousal plus thoughts of avoidance, anger therefore is arousal plus thoughts of attacking. Try Exercise 31.

Reflect on one or more times when you were angry. Note the Antecedent, Behaviour and Consequences. The word antecedent is taken to mean events leading to the behaviour, this could be anything from being shouted at to missing your bus. Behaviour in this context is taken to mean the action which one performs as a result of being angry. Consequence is basically the outcome, that is, what was the result of being angry. Say for example, the antecedent, behaviour and consequences of my anger were:

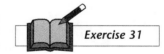

Exercise 31

- Antecedent. Another driver flashed his lights continuously to suggest that I let him through
- Behaviour. I responded negatively, that is I stayed where I was and did not let him pass
- Consequence. The driver appeared frustrated and showed numerous rude gestures and tried to drive bumper to bumper with my car.

It might be an idea to discuss your findings with one of your colleagues. The whole purpose of this exercise is to make the point that anger is a natural emotion and as such one should be encouraged to express it whenever and wherever possible. It might also be an idea to check out what is the most common event which makes you angry. Wallbott and Scherer's (1989) study showed the most common antecedents of anger to be

- problems with relationships
- interactions with strangers
- injustice and
- inconveniences

One learns through socialisation, to ignore the warning that anger brings, instead one chooses to view it as a weakness or a bad thing. Anger is often mistakenly seen as a negative emotion, sometimes it is referred to as inappropriate in the sense that nobody wants to know when someone is angry. Having said that, society is gradually coming to terms with the fact that anger is a normal aspect of one's life. Anger suggests a strong feeling of annoyance. When people are angry, they lose their rationality and function purely from an emotional dimension. The individual exhibits a variety of behaviour from mild irritation to destruction.

Make a list of the ways you behave when you are angry.

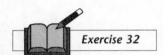 *Exercise 32*

Now reflect on your list and decide whether the things that you do fall into either the Acceptable or Unacceptable category.

Discuss this with a colleague. This would be quite interesting in that what is acceptable to you may not be acceptable to your colleague.

Although strictly speaking anger is very much an intrapersonal element, it is mostly expressed in overt behaviour, that is, in aggression. Having said that, it needs to be stressed that people can deal with their own anger in one of three ways and these are:

1   Anger Expressed Outward (for example in destructive behaviour); violent behaviour directed at other people or things is an example of anger out. The Dunblane massacre would be one such example.
2   Anger Expressed Inward (usually seen in depression); suicide or attempted suicide.
3   Anger Repressed or Suppressed (here it is as if the anger feeling is placed on hold).

Anger which is expressed inward or repressed/suppressed would fall into the category of maladaptive behaviour. Anger expressed outward can also be categorised as maladaptive if it is exhibited as uncontrolled aggression. If on the other hand aggression is diverted through the correct channel, as in boxing, it would be seen as an adaptive behaviour. Stearns and Stearns (1986, p.2) remarked, 'Americans today worry about their emotions more . . . . .than most Victorians husbands, ever did. And there is no emotion about which we fret, amid greater confusion, than anger. While our founding fathers felt relatively free to storm and rage when the mood seized them and even took temper to be a sign of manliness, we have become embarrassed by such display today.' It would be wrong to believe that this particular sentiment is related solely to the Americans. One is inclined to believe that anger is seen as a negative emotion with a clear message that it should be repressed.

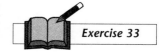

Theories of anger

Plutchik (1994) believed that when one thinks of a specific event which triggers anger, one also recognises that people can sometimes appear to be angry or irritable most of the time, regardless of the situations which they find themselves in. These people are usually described as having a personality trait of anger.

Perhaps you could pause and think of some of the people you know who would fit into this category. I am sure some of you will recall Steve Wright's fictitious character, 'Mr Angry' on BBC Radio 1, *Coronation Street's* Jim MacDonald or *Eastenders'* The Mitchell Brothers.

Exercise 33

Psychoanalytical theory of anger

There are various psychological theories which attempt to offer some understanding as to why a person becomes angry. The main argument seems to be based on the nature versus nurture debate. From Freud's dual instinct theory, Eros and Thanatos, one can deduce that all those powerful emotions are like hydraulic energy and as the energy increases within the person, the latter is motivated towards its discharge. Eros is the life instinct and this is displayed in the form of sexual energy. Thanatos on the other hand is the instinct of death and its motivation is geared towards death and destruction. The expression of Thanatos is through aggressive behaviour. The instinct of aggression is aroused through frustration of the Id. The aggressive energy according to Freud, must be externalised in order to protect the individual from self-harm. From this perspective therefore the argument is that aggression is innate, that is the individual is born with it.

Frustration–aggression hypothesis

Dollard *et al.* (1939) claimed that all aggression results from an experience of frustration. People basically become frustrated if they are blocked from reaching their goals. This in turn initiates anger which produces an aggressive drive and leads to aggressive behaviour. Dollard *et al.*'s theory became known as the 'Frustration–Aggression Hypothesis' where aggression is always seen as a result of frustration. This sentiment is also reflected in Abraham Maslow's writings (discussed in Chapter 6).

Social learning theory

According to Bandura (1973), aggression, like most behaviour, is a learned behaviour. Learning is facilitated by role models. The social learning theory suggests that learning occurs through reinforcement, direct observation and instruction.

Reinforcement of behaviour

Reinforcement of behaviour is based on the principles of operant conditioning (discussed in Chapter 11) and suggests that if a behaviour, in this case anger, displayed through aggression, is rewarded then the behaviour will persist. Let us take bullying as an aggressive behaviour. According to the principles of operant conditioning, the persecutor or oppressor is rewarded through perhaps feeling in total control or through material gain, over the victim. The aggressive behaviour will become more persistent.

Direct observation

Direct observation suggests that if children observe aggressive behaviour exhibited by others, there is a strong possibility that they will show aggressive behaviour. Bandura's (1973) study showed that observing aggressive models greatly increases the amount of aggressive display in children's behaviour. The study involved a group of nursery school children watching a film during which an adult expressed different forms of aggressive behaviour toward an inflated Bobo doll. The result of the study showed that these children imitated many of the aggressive behaviours which they had observed from watching the film. Some have argued that the tragic death of Jamie Bulger is linked to the phenomenon of observational learning of violent movies such as *Child's Play*.

Instruction

Instruction suggests an element of 'being told what to do'. Bandura and Walters (1959) showed that parents of aggressive male adolescents are more inclined to urge their boys to stand up for their rights and are actively involved in shaping their children's aggressive behaviour.

Functions of anger and aggression

Ventilation of anger

Although in many ways aggression can be seen as a negative expression of anger, it has to be said that aggression serves a definite purpose in life. Jackson (1954) stated that the source of aggression is anger and its aim is to destroy the object which is responsible for the arousal of anger. For example I feel angry when someone shouts racial abuse at me, in turn I curse and swear at him. The act of cursing and swearing serves to vent my feelings, although rude, it nevertheless makes me feel better and my anger dissipates.

Defence against anxiety

According to Sullivan (1953), people behave aggressively in order to deal with their own anxieties in an attempt to protect themselves, as though neutralising the anxiety provoking situation. 'If I can show you that I can be as violent as you then there is little chance that you'll carry on threatening me (this is conditional on my physical strength of course).'

Controlling function

Aggression is also used to dominate or to exert total control over someone else. The notion of 'Let them know who is boss' would fit this category. If for example I behave aggressively, no one will dare to tread on my toe, and hence the controlling element.

Protective function

The protective function is very much based on the principle of defence against a hostile enemy. I display aggressive behaviour to warn the enemy that I am not an easy prey. This is somewhat similar to the controlling function.

Pause and reflect on how you deal with your own anger. Discuss this with your group.

Reflect on how you deal with other people's anger (let the other people include your patients or clients) and again discuss this with your group.

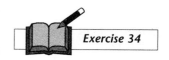

Exercise 34

Emotion and the concept of caring

In many ways emotion can be seen as an integral part of communication and it is revealed through the expressive aspect (mainly facial) of one's behaviour. According to Rogers (1951), therapeutic communication can only be enhanced if there is an element of transparency on the part of the caregiver. This means that the caregiver's behaviour needs to be congruent with his or her feelings. Having said this, one needs to bear in mind that this may not always be appropriate. When this is the case then it would be much more beneficial for both the patient and carer, if the latter does not engage in the helping process. At least that way the carer does not have to adopt a pseudo-caring role, which in the long run can be harmful to both parties. Awareness of the nature of one's emotion therefore holds the key to a good rapport and a positive attitude towards one's patient. Attitudes and prejudices are the topics of Chapter 8.

References

Armon-Jones, C. (1986). The social functions of emotion. In: Harre, R. (Ed.) *The Social Constructions of Emotions*. Basil Blackwell.

Bandura, A. (1973). *Aggression: A Social Learning Analysis*. Englewood Cliffs, NJ: Prentice Hall.

Bandura, A. and Walters, R.H. (1959). *Adolescent Aggression*. New York: Ronald.

Delgado, J.M.R. (1971). *Physical Control of the Mind: Toward a Psychocivilized Society*. New York: Harper and Row.

Dollard, J., Doob, L.W., Miller, N.E., Mowrer, O.H. and Sears, R.R. (1939). *Frustration and Aggression*. New Haven, CT: Yale University Press.

Harre, R. (Ed.) (1986). *The Social Constructions of Emotions*. Oxford: Basil Blackwell.

Izard, C.E. (1977). *Human Emotion*. New York, London: Plenum Press.

Jackson, L. (1954). *Aggression and its Interpretation*. London: Methuen.

Plutchik, R. (1984). 'Emotions: A general psychoevolutionary theory.' In: Scherer, K.R. and Ekman, P. (Eds) *Approaches to Emotion*. London: Lawrence Erlbaum Associates.

Plutchik, R. and Kellerman, H. (1980). (Eds) *Emotion: Theory, Research and Experience: Vol. 1. Theories of Emotion*. New York: Academic Press.

Plutchik, R. (1994). *The Psychology and Biology of Emotion*. Harper Collins College Publishers.

Rogers, C.R. (1951). *Client Centred Therapy*. London: Constable.

Stearns, C.Z. and Stearns, P.N. (1986). *Anger: The Struggle for Emotional Control in America's History*. Chicago, London: University of Chicago Press.

Sullivan, H.S. (1953). *The Interpersonal Theory of Psychiatry*. New York: W.W. Norton.

Wallbott, H.G. and Scherer, K.R. (1989). 'Assessing emotion by questionnaire.' In: Plutchik, R. and Kellerman, H. (Eds) *Emotion: Theory, Research and Experience: Vol 4: The Measurement of Emotions*. New York: Academic Press.

Attitudes and prejudices 8

Objectives

After reading this chapter you should be able to:

1   Define attitude and prejudices
2   Describe the components of both attitudes and prejudice
3   Identify the functions of attitudes
4   Explain how attitude and prejudice are formed
5   Describe how attitude can be changed
6   Describe the link between attitude, values and belief
7   Recognise and accept your own prejudice
8   Explain how a knowledge of attitude and prejudice can enhance care delivery

There is a consensus of opinion to suggest that attitudes, values and beliefs are abstract concepts which are intertwined. Each has a direct influence on the other two. Each of these concepts are explored separately here and the starting point is with attitude.

Attitudes

Allport (1935) defined an attitude as a mental state of readiness which is organised through experience and it exerts a direct influence on people's response to all objects to which it is related. A mental state of readiness suggests that attitude is not a behaviour. This means that it is not something that one can observe. Having said that one can see the behaviour people exhibit as a result of their attitude but not the attitude itself. Oskamp (1991) explains that it is a preparation for a certain behaviour, for example it prepares me to respond in a particular way to the object toward which my attitude is aimed. Object is taken to include people, things, action and situation. This mental state of readiness is based on past and present experience and it gives direction and guidance to the response. The nature of attitudes can be seen to have three components and these are

- cognitive
- affective and
- behavioural

Cognitive component

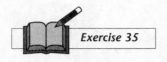

Exercise 35

The cognitive component of attitude is described as a belief or idea that the person has about an object. Say for example in this particular context the objects in question are patients.

Make a very brief statement of your belief or idea about patients. What or who do you think patients are? Whatever statement you come up with, that would be the cognitive component of your attitude. This is basically your opinions, ideas, and impressions about the object of your attitude.

Affective component

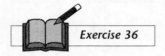

Exercise 36

The affective component of attitude is described as the emotions and feelings which are aroused towards the object of one's attitude. In our case the object of our attitude is the patients. Here again have a go at Exercise 36.

Write a brief statement about your emotion/feeling about patients. What do you feel about patients? Or to put it another way, how do patients make you feel?

The statement you come up with is the affective component of your attitude.

Behavioural component

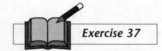

Exercise 37

This is described as one's action towards the object of one's attitude.

Following on from the last two exercises what action could you take? What would or could you do for patients?

Whatever action you take this would be seen as the behavioural component of your attitude towards patients.

Let me try and put this in context and for the sake of argument let the brief statements of my cognitive, affective and behavioural components be as follows:

I believe that more could be done to raise patients' quality of care (cognitive).
I feel sad and depressed about patients' standard of care (affective).
I could campaign actively for more resources thus ensuring patients have a better deal (behavioural).

The scenario that has been offered also shows the interactions which exist between all these components, it is basically I think, I feel and I act.

Functional aspects of attitude

Obviously one holds different attitudes towards different objects. The individual may feel positive about certain things and negative about others. Some theorists would argue that one's attitudes serve specific purposes. This basically means that there may be a well-defined goal for one's attitudes, one may be conscious or unconscious of such a goal. Both Katz (1960) and McGuire (1969) share similar ideas about the functional aspects of attitudes and for simplicity the focus will be on the four reasons McGuire has highlighted. These are as follows.

1   Utilitarian or adaptive function
2   Ego-defence function
3   Economy or knowledge function
4   Value-expressive function

Utilitarian or adaptive function

The utilitarian function basically means that people hold a certain attitude because it is held by the majority of the members of a group and if they want to remain a member of that group then they have no choice but to hold the same attitude as the rest of the members of the group. It is more like a question of changing or modifying one's attitudes to fit in. The Tetley bitter advertisement sums up the utilitarian or adaptive function succinctly, 'If you can't beat them, join them'. Perhaps it would be true to say that this particular function of attitudes is commonly shared by almost everyone at some time or other. This may have been a conscious or an unconscious phenomenon.

Reflect, recall and note one or two of your attitudes which may have a utilitarian or adaptive purpose.

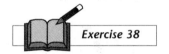
Exercise 38

Here are some common ones:
Friends smoke therefore I do
I dress in a certain style to fit in
I wear a suit and tie at a job interview to be accepted

Ego defensive function

The defensive function of attitudes basically protect people from acknowledging certain basic truths about themselves or about certain realities of the world. Oskamp (1991, p.76) argues that everyone uses defence mechanisms to some extent, 'but they are used much more by individuals who are insecure or feel inferior or who have deep internal conflicts'. The concept of mental defence mechanism is discussed in Chapter 2 and here perhaps you may wish to consider Exercise 39.

Reflect and recall on any ego defence function of the attitudes you may have displayed.

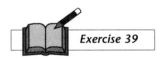
Exercise 39

You may if you wish look for your own examples of denial, displacement or projection, introjection and suppression if these are applicable.

Economy or knowledge function

The economy or knowledge function of attitudes tends to help people to understand and make sense of what is going on around them. Attitudes give one information about a certain object, for example one could say that politicians only tell the truth if it suits them.

Value-expressive function

Some would argue that the value-expressive function allows people to demonstrate an attitude which is appropriate to their personal values and to their self-concepts. Some examples are:

*   wearing Mohican hairstyle
*   wearing nose studs or in the case of Spice girl Mel B, on the tongue

- wearing one's hair yellow or purple
- wearing a Leeds or Liverpool football shirt
- waving the British flag at the European games

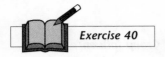

Exercise 40

Reflect and list some of the things that you do which may fit into the value-expressive function of attitude.

Formation of attitude

The phrase 'attitude formation' means the birth of one's attitude about an object. One could basically say that no attitude about that particular object existed prior to its formation. It is easier to conceptualise attitude formation in the world of an infant. One could argue that an infant is born without attitudes and these are formed as the child develops his or her schema. It is much more difficult to see an adult as having no attitude, although this may well be the case. 'For adults to have no attitude may mean that they have never had any experience, either direct or vicarious, with the object . . . or simply that they have never thought evaluatively about it' (Oskamp, 1991, p.154). Attitude change is quite different and it implies that the attitude is present and that for one reason or another it alters. Attitude formation and attitude change can be seen as having similar processes in terms of their development and for this particular reason these terms will be used interchangeably.

Attitude formation or change can be said to take place through:

1   Direct experience
2   Parental influence
3   Group influence
4   Media influence

Direct experience

Direct experience or exposure means being in personal contact with the object of one's attitude. Oskamp (1991, p.158) states that this is 'the earliest and the most fundamental way in which people form attitudes'. Attitudes which are formed through direct exposure are said to be stronger in intensity and permanency. Direct experience suggests an element of being actually involved, as in 'been there and done it'. I had a go at parascending and liked it, that would be my direct experience with the object (parascending) of my attitude. Personal or direct experience can be viewed from two aspects:

- Salient Incidents. These include traumas, fears and other critical events during one's life.
- Repeated Exposure. These include the constant bombardment by advertisers or political parties, in their attempts to change people's attitudes to either buy their products or to vote for them.

Parental influence

Here perhaps lies the most influential factor in attitude formation. Oskamp argues that a child's attitudes are largely shaped by its own experience with the world but much of that experience is influenced by parental attitudes. If attitudes are viewed as schemas, as suggested by Eagly and Chaiken (1993), then parental influences cannot be underestimated. By its very definition schema is a cognitive map or mould for processing information, therefore who is better placed to shape this mould than parents?

The impact of group influence on attitudes is as important as parental influence. Group influence would include schools and peers. Health care education could in fact be regarded as an attitude-changing process. Teachers are one of the most influential groups of people responsible for changing one's attitudes. Peer groups have similar influences especially through peer pressures.

Group influence

The impact of learning on attitude

Classical, operant and social learning theories offer valuable contributions to clarifying the concept of attitude formation and attitude change. Watson and Rayner (1920) used the principles of classical conditioning to change Little Albert's positive attitude towards a white rat into a negative attitude (see Section II, Chapter 11). In the same way people can be conditioned consciously or unconsciously to hold either positive or negative attitudes towards any object. Ajzen (1993) says that generally speaking people form beliefs about an object by associating it with certain attributes, as for example with other objects or events. In Little Albert's case the situation was deliberately manipulated to achieve the desired result, in reality however conditioning goes on all the time whether one is aware of it or not. Listed below are some of the instances where classical conditioning would have been at play.

Attitude and classical learning

- Fear of dentists
- Fear of hospitals
- Fear of doctors
- Negative thoughts or feelings towards foreigners
- Negative thoughts or feelings towards people with mental health problems
- Negative thoughts or feelings towards people with learning disabilities
- Negative views towards old people
- Negative views towards youths
- Negative impression of a patient whose breath smells of alcohol
- Fear of homosexuals (both males and females)

Try and see if you can link some of your attitudes to the principles of classical conditioning. See also if you can explain those listed in terms of conditioned, unconditioned stimulus and response. I will start you off with fear of dentists, see Figure 8.1.

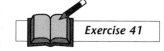

Exercise 41

Let us assume that an individual starts with a neutral or positive attitude towards dentists. People go to their dentists and undergo treatment which involves the usual cleaning, drilling, injection, filling, and possible extraction. Initially their attitude toward dentists is positive or at least neutral. The treatment however, by its very nature causes pain and generates fear through their reflexive properties. The repeated visits to the dentist lead to a gradual association of the pain and or fear with the person (dentist), until eventually at the mere mention of the word dentist, the individual is filled with horror. His/her attitude toward the dentist changes from positive to negative. This attitude could also be generalised towards all dentists. Although this is a very simplistic illustration of how classical conditioning can alter people's attitude, nevertheless it has to be said that it is very powerful, especially so when one's sexual and emotional feelings are targeted. Most of the advertisements for example are based on this principle. Usually a sexually attractive person (Nicole) is paired with the product (Renault Clio) and this association helps in the formation of one's positive attitude regarding that product. A local newspaper headline reads, "Nicole is tres bien at spreading the message." Willard (1996) states that Nicole and Papa have done more for the Renault Clio than the most persuasive salesperson who can memorise every technical fact and finance package. The result of this particular advertisement has meant an approximate 200,000 Clios in Britain. Now imagine what would happen if it was drilled into your head that if the members of some ethnic groups were to move into your locality, house prices in that locality would depreciate, or that these ethnic groups would do you out of a job.

Nicole and Papa

Attitude and operant conditioning

Section II, Chapter 11 discusses the principle of operant conditioning, here however suffice it to say that its main focus is on positive and negative reward reinforcing behaviour and punishment eradicates unwanted behaviour. If, for example, a teacher praises a pupil, he/she is more likely to enjoy the subject, if a teacher gives minimal homework (homework is taken to be the aversive or painful stimulus) the chances are the pupil will like the subject, but if on the other hand the teacher punishes the pupil through detentions or any other means, the pupil will learn to detest the subject.

Self-awareness and attitude

How aware are people of their attitudes? The simple answer is, not at all. From an attitude point of view, people tend to function in an unconscious mode. In some instances being aware of one's attitudes may be too painful especially since one may need to confront and change them. It is safer to believe that what one thinks, feels and does, is right. The problem is always with the other person, never with oneself. The sad truth however, is that the problem is with every individual. The thought that one could be jealous and envious of others, is too painful to feel, acknowledging it therefore can be too traumatic an experience to endure. People are very good at critically observing the attitudes of others and expressing their dislikes at what they find. Let us be adventurous and explore our own attitudes. Have a go at Exercise 42.

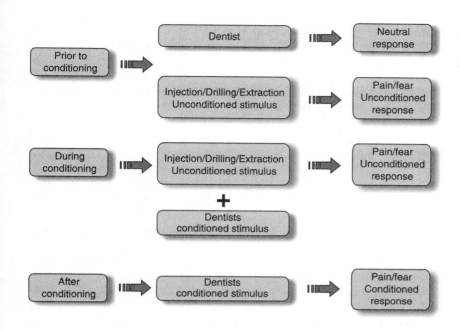

Figure 8.1
The sequence of classical conditioning and the fear of dentists

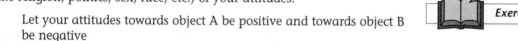

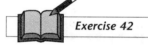

Choose two objects (A and B, these could be people or any topic you choose like religion, politics, sex, race, etc.) of your attitudes.

Exercise 42

- Let your attitudes towards object A be positive and towards object B be negative
- You can chose to identify your objects if you wish
- Make a list of your behaviour towards both these objects
- Now reflect on both your behaviour and ask yourself, 'why do or did I behave this way'
- Make a list of your possible reasons
- Select your most honest reason and decide whether it was the object of your attitude (people, things, or environment) or your attitude itself which is the result of your behaviour
- You may chose to discuss this with a friend or colleague

Values

According to Rokeach (1968) a value is an important life goal or societal condition which is desired by a person. Value can be both abstract and concrete. Values like peace, justice, freedom, beauty, life and happiness are seen as abstract. Money and other material things on the other hand are seen as concrete. Oskamp (1991, p.13) states, 'values are ends rather than means – the goals a person strives to reach rather than the methods (s)he uses to get there'. By its very own nature values can only be positive, for example if I say I value truth, this would suggest that I see truth as positive and that I would relate positively to people who are truthful. Values are seen as the central core to one's attitude in that it influences many of one's attitudes and beliefs.

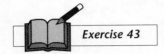

Exercise 43

List some of your values and note their special significance for you. Discuss these with a friend or colleague.

Beliefs

Fishbein and Ajzen (1975) define beliefs as statements which indicate a person's subjective probability that an object has a particular characteristic. Unlike attitudes, which are tri-components in nature, beliefs are purely cognitive. Beliefs are referred to as ideas and thoughts, the contents of which can be described as true or false, 'correct or incorrect; evaluate it as good or bad; or advocate a certain course of action or certain state of existence as desirable or undesirable' (Rokeach, 1970, p.13).

Beliefs are seen to have three dimensions and these are descriptive, evaluative and prescriptive.

Descriptive beliefs

Descriptive beliefs offer information about the object of one's beliefs. For example I could say, I believe that London is approximately 200 miles from Leeds.

Evaluative beliefs

Evaluative beliefs offer a judgement on the object of one's belief. For example I believe that Manchester United is the richest football team in this country.

Prescriptive beliefs

Prescriptive beliefs reflect the sentiments of a request or demand on the object of one's belief. I could say that I believe that nurses should be more assertive in order to fulfil the role of patients' advocate.

Thus far the example of beliefs that have been offered are somewhat superficial. In order to fit this in the context of your own beliefs, try the exercise below.

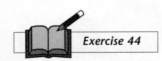

Exercise 44

Write a few short statements of your beliefs about the following.

- Mental and physical health
- Your profession
- Politics

You may if you wish, share and discuss these with your colleagues.

Prejudice

Do we really understand the concept of prejudice? Better still do we recognise our own prejudices? We all would like to stamp out prejudice and yet we unconsciously carry around the very germ of prejudice which contaminates our very own existence.

'Of all human weaknesses, none is more destructive of the dignity of the individual and the social bonds of humanity than prejudice' (Zimbardo, 1992, p.599). Perhaps it would be true to say that this is one weakness which has escaped one's awareness. Prejudice is seen as a characteristic which can only be attributed to others, reality however suggests that every individual is guilty of being prejudiced. In a sense it is more like an insidious disease rather than a weakness. A disease which is cleverly repressed within one's invisible self and the camouflage is so perfect that the individual is left believing that he or she is not prejudiced. I may be doing some of you an injustice, but my general belief is that we would all like to believe and feel that we are not prejudiced but should we be found guilty of being prejudiced, then let it be in favour of someone or something but never against anyone. Bethlehem (1985, p.2) had this to say, 'one can be prejudiced in favour of black Englishmen, as well as against them; and one's prejudices can concern motor cars and tinned soup as well as ethnic groups. I suspect that I, and many other social psychologists, are prejudiced against people we classify as "racists".' It would not be an exaggeration therefore to say that there is no escape, we are all guilty of being prejudiced, some of us are perhaps guiltier than others.

Allport (1958) defined prejudice as an aversive or hostile attitude towards a person who belongs to a group simply because he belongs to that group. Harding *et al.* (1969) on the other hand believe that prejudice is an intolerant, unfair, or irrational unfavourable attitude towards another group of people. Although both these definitions clearly imply a negative and an undesirable flavour to the sentiment of prejudice, nevertheless it has to be said that prejudice can be positive, for example the French are romantic, Italian men are seen as great lovers, the British are dependable and the Japanese are industrious. When the subject of prejudice is brought up however, it is always discussed in its negative form. This chapter is a case in point.

Tri-dimensional aspects of prejudice

The three-dimensional aspects of prejudice are similar to that of attitude, these are cognitive, affective and behavioural.

The affective component of prejudice seems to be the most dominant part, and it even influences the cognition to such an extent that it interferes with logic reasoning, thus creating an imbalance between these two components (see Figure 8.2). Pettigrew *et al.* (1982) state that numerous emotions are involved in prejudice and these include; 'fear and threat, or jealousy and envy; it can range from intense hatred to simple indifference and absence of human sympathy' (p.14). It needs to be pointed out here that if one is to take it that there is a positive side to prejudice then what must follow is the positive display of affect. This could include extreme admiration and love.

Affective component of prejudice

Pettigrew *et al.* (1982, p.5) explain that in an attempt to make sense of our chaotic universe, which is bombarded with more sensory stimulation than we can possibly process and use, we strive 'to organise the environment and give it meaning by simplifying and packaging the incoming stimuli into readily useful information'. In doing so however people make mistakes and these have significant effects on their prejudice. One such

Cognitive component of prejudice

mistake is the concept of stereotyping. Stereotyping is seen to be powerful and dangerous because it involves false interpretation that all the members of an outgroup share the same characteristics, for example Blacks are lazy, Jews are shrewd, and Pakistanis are dirty. Here again one has to consider that such a misconception of any group can turn out to be positive to fit in with positive stereotyping, such as, Italian men are great lovers.

Behavioural component of prejudice

The behavioural component of prejudice includes any discriminatory act which ranges from racial jokes, verbal hostility, physical attack to actual genocide as in the case of Nazi Germany against the Jews.

There is a constant interplay between attitude and prejudice and perhaps it would be better to explore this before going any further.

Say for example one is positively prejudiced towards a group of people. Close analysis of the dynamics of prejudice would reveal favourable cognition, affect and behaviour towards that particular group of people. It could be argued that one of the cognitive aspects of prejudice is stereotyping (see Figure 8.2). Pettigrew *et al.* (1982) define stereotyping as an overgeneralisation of psychological characteristics to large human groups. In this instance, suppose that the generalisation is favourable to Italian men. Despite being a favourable notion, the fact remains that it is still a misconception to believe that all Italian men are great lovers. The affective outcome of this stereotypic impression of Italian men is bound to be favourable too. Women therefore will feel good to be with Italian men, and will have great esteem for them. Some may admire them while others may fall in love with them. This leads to the behavioural aspect of prejudice. Some women may in fact date or even marry Italian men and everyone lives happily ever after.

Unfortunately the darker side of prejudice never has a happy ending. Here right from the start the picture is doom and gloom. Again let the starting point be cognitive, the stereotypic image of all Pakistanis is that they are dirty and smelly. This arouses a negative set of feelings and emotions, which can range from disgust to repulsion. The behaviour which may follow can take various forms from verbal hostility to actual physical attacks and even murders.

Figure 8.2
The tri-dimensional aspects of prejudice and its corollaries

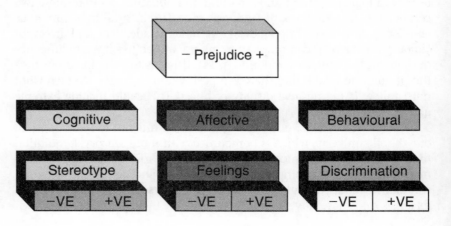

We all know that in one way or another, we are all prejudiced. The question is, what is the nature of our prejudices? Bearing in mind that a prejudice can be defined as an attitude towards any object or situation, based purely on emotion and a faulty cognition, list some of your prejudices. The aim here is to recognise and acknowledge one's own prejudices, it is not necessary therefore to discuss your prejudices with anyone.

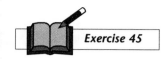

Exercise 45

Being prejudice or not being prejudice is not the question, because it is clear that we all are. The question is 'to what extent are we prejudiced?' In case you are experiencing some difficulty in being able to recall any of your prejudices, perhaps the concept of cognitive set will help.

Prejudiced or not prejudiced that is not the question

Cognitive set

Cognitive set can be described as blinkered thought. This means that one's thoughts are restricted to viewing people's behaviour according to a set of criteria, which is defined by commonly held perceptions. And here is a 'this really happened to me' scenario.

'One Thursday morning an engineer was due to call to service our central heating. As soon as I returned home from work, I asked my wife, 'Was he here then?' 'No' my wife replied, 'He wasn't, but *she* was and *she* did a very good job too.'

It never at that moment, crossed my mind that the engineer could be a woman and ashamedly I had to admit to suffering from a cognitive set. I hasten to add that there are others who perhaps still believe that doctors and surgeons are men, nurses are women, similarly a manager is a man and a secretary is a woman. Some would argue that there is a very thin line between cognitive set and prejudice. If you truly want to know whether you are prejudiced or not, try this simple but very common exercise.

- Step 1: Choose any group of people you want as long as they are of a different ethnic origin to yourself.
- Step 2: Construct a social distance scale starting with a statement of the type of relationship you would find acceptable, for example:

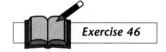

Exercise 46

I would find it acceptable for (a person within your chosen group) to:

1.	Visit my country	Yes/No
2.	Reside in my country	Yes/No
3.	Work in the same department as myself	Yes/No
4.	Be my co-worker	Yes/No
5.	Live in my locality	Yes/No
6.	Live in the same street	Yes/No
7.	Have lunch or a drink with me	Yes/No
8.	Be my neighbour	Yes/No
9.	Be my close friend	Yes/No
10.	Marry or become involved with members of my family	Yes/No

- Step 3: If you want to know about any other group of people even those of the same origin as yourself, all you have to do is to substitute the group in brackets above and repeat Step 2. Example of groups could include:

People with mental health problems
Homosexual (lesbians and gays)
People who are dependent on drugs, alcohol etc.
Unemployed
Old people
Fat people
Black people

From point 6 onward you will find it much more difficult to decide and perhaps you could surprise yourself to discover the true nature of your intrapersonal dynamics.

Stockwell's concept of the unpopular patient

Stockwell (1984) surprised many in the nursing profession with her concept of the 'Unpopular Patient'. Prior to the publication of her research, the majority of nurses were not aware that they could in fact be prejudiced towards patients. Stockwell showed that there are key contributory factors which determine whether a nurse enjoys caring for patients or not. For example those patients who 'communicated readily with nurses, knew the nurses' name, were able to joke and laugh with the nurses and co-operated in being helped to get well and expressed determination to do so' (Stockwell, 1984, p.46), were perceived as enjoyable to care for. Those who were not enjoyable to care for, included patients who indicated that they were not happy being in the ward or with what was being done for them, by grumbling and complaining or otherwise demanding attention and those whom the nurses felt did not need to be in hospital, or should not be in that particular ward. This is not dissimilar to a lecturer's idea of what a good student is. If the student is compliant, and attends every lesson and never asks difficult questions and is always polite, he or she will be perceived as the best. Attitude and prejudice are perhaps two of the most influential factors which actually guide care delivery. This implies that lack of awareness of one's attitude can be catastrophic for the recipients of care. The best protection against negative attitude and prejudice is the caregiver's own self-awareness. Self-awareness will in fact reflect the carer's particular vantage point, which in turn will guide effective care.

How a knowledge of attitude and prejudice can enhance health care delivery

Learn to respect people's attitude because they have their own individuality and uniqueness. Their attitude may be dictated by their own culture or religion.

Attitude serves a particular purpose and by exploring some of the functions of attitude, the helper may be able to establish the 'why' of a patient's behaviour.

Attitude is about one's own likes and dislikes; it helps the carer to see it from the patient's own particular perspective.

The helper can in fact predict patient's behaviour – for example if someone says life is not worth living, this can provide cues about his/her mental health state and precautions can be taken to protect the patient from self-harm.

Exploring the components of attitude (cognitive, affective and behavioural) may explain people's aversion towards hospitals, doctors, nurses and medication.

The carer's knowledge of attitude is seen as crucial to the enhancement of health care delivery. Many more issues can be added to the above list through group discussion or brain-storming sessions. Attitude in the form of prejudice is one of those intrapersonal dynamics which is firmly imbedded in one's emotions. Although it may be very difficult to change, awareness of the helper's own attitude is a prerequisite to caring.

References

Ajzen, I. (1993). 'Attitude theory and the attitude-behaviour relation.' In: Krebs, D. and Schmidt, P. (Eds) *New Directions in Attitude Measurement*. New York: Walter de Gruyter.

Allport, G. (1935). 'Attitudes.' In: Murchison, C. (Ed.) *Handbook of Social Psychology*. Worcester, MA: Clark University Press, pp. 798–844.

Allport, G.W. (1958). *The Nature of Prejudice*. New York: Dounleuay Anchor Books, Doubleday and Company.

Bethlehem, D.W. (1985). *A Social Psychology of Prejudice*. London: Croom Helm.

Eagly, A.H. and Chaiken, S. (1993). *The Psychology of Attitudes*. London: Harcourt Brace Jovanovich College Publishers.

Fishbein, M. and Ajzen, I. (1975). *Belief, Attitude, Intention and Behaviour: An Introduction to Theory and Research*. Reading, MA: Addison-Wesley.

Harding, J., Proshawsky, H., Kutner, B. and Chein, I. (1969). 'Prejudice and ethnic relations.' In: Lindzey, G. and Aronson, E. (Eds) *The Handbook of Social Psychology*, 2nd edn, Vol. 5, Reading, MA: Addison-Wesley, pp. 1–76.

Katz, D. (1960). 'The functional approach to the study of attitudes.' *Public Opinion Quarterly*, **24**, 163–204.

McGuire, W.J. (1969). 'The nature of attitudes and attitude change.' In: Lindzey, G. and Aronson, E. (Eds) *The Handbook of Social Psychology*, 2nd edn, Vol. 3, Reading, MA: Addison-Wesley, pp. 136–314.

Oskamp, S. (1991). *Attitudes and Opinions*. Englewood Cliffs, NJ: Prentice Hall.

Pettigrew, T.F., Fredrickson, G.M., Knobel, D.T., Glazer, N. and Ueda, R. (1982). *Prejudice: Dimensions of Ethnicity*. Cambridge, MA, London, England: The Belknap Press of Harvard University Press.

Rokeach, M. (1968). *Beliefs, Attitudes, and Values. A Theory of Organisation and Change.* San Francisco: Jossey-Bass.

Rokeach, M. (1970). *Beliefs, Attitudes, and Values: A Theory of Organisation and Change.* San Francisco: Jossey-Bass.

Stockwell, F. (1984). *The Unpopular Patient.* London: RCN.

Watson, J.B. and Rayner, R. (1920). 'Conditioned emotional reactions.' *Journal of Experimental Psychology*, 3, 1–14.

Willard, T. (1996). 'Nicole is tres bien at spreading the message.' *Observer* (local) Midweek. No. 127. 3 September.

Zimbardo, P. (1992). *Psychology of Life.* New York: Harper Collins.

Interpersonal dynamics and self-awareness

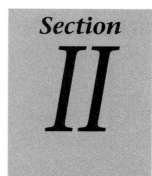

Introduction

The focus throughout Section I has been on some of those intrapersonal dynamics, which are the loci of meaning. Although it was argued that the sources of behaviour rest from within, nevertheless one has to say that one's knowledge of people's behaviour can be further enhanced by observing them in action. Action is taken to mean both what one says and what one does. These are embraced in the realm of interpersonal behaviour. Myers and Myers (1992, p.7), define interpersonal communication as a transaction between people and their environment. Interpersonal behaviour therefore can be described as a transaction between two or more individuals, who are acting and reacting to each other in turn. Interpersonal behaviour processes are those behaviours which one can see, hear and feel. It could be argued that interpersonal interaction is the pivot in the existence of life. It is a need and a necessity. The variety of interpersonal communication ranges from people who are intimate with one another to people who are total strangers. The emphasis of this section is on those observable behaviours. Having said that, it is beyond the scope of this book to deal with all observable behaviour, the focus therefore will be on some of those behaviours which are considered to be significant to the health care professions. These include:

- Coping strategies
- Obedience
- Conformity
- Compliance
- Group dynamics
- Leadership, leadership styles and
- Conflicts

The starting point of this part is with the works of Harry Stack Sullivan (1953) and Erik Erikson (1963). Both Sullivan and Erikson demonstrated clearly the significant role of the environment as plausible rationale for why people behave the way they do. The word environment is taken to include people and objects. Sullivan's theory (1953) is called the

Interpersonal Theory of Psychiatry. This however does not mean that his entire focus is on people with mental health problems. On the contrary, the emphasis is on anxiety as a tension which impinges on the human organism. This human organism could be any one of us. Erikson on the other hand made growth and development the basic foundation for his psychosocial theory. The theory is called psychosocial because of the constant interaction between people and their environment throughout growth and development.

References

Erikson, H. (1963). *Childhood and Society*. New York: Norton.

Myers, G.E. and Myers, M.T. (1992). *The Dynamics of Human Communication: A Laboratory Approach*. London: McGraw-Hill.

Sullivan, H.S. (1953). *The Interpersonal Theory of Psychiatry*. New York: Norton.

Interpersonal theory

9

Objectives

After reading this chapter you should be able to:

1 Describe some of the major points of Sullivan's interpersonal theory such as:
   a One's need for satisfaction and security,
   b One's way of dealing with fear,
   c The Self system and
   d The stages of personality development
2 Explain some of the strategies an individual may employ in transaction with others

Sullivan's (1892–1949) interpersonal theory of personality development

Sullivan's (1953) focus was on interpersonal processes that could be observed in social settings. Sullivan believed that people can get to know more about others by actually observing them interacting with one another. The energising forces of behaviour rest with two prime motivating factors and these are:

- The need for satisfaction
- The need for security

The need for satisfaction

It would seem that, right from an early age, as young as babies, people are in search of satisfaction of their needs, and these include their biological needs, for example food, water, sleep and sex. There are two forces which act against each other and Sullivan called these Absolute Euphoria and Absolute Tension. Absolute euphoria is defined as a state of utter well being. Sullivan (1953) argued that the nearest approach to this 'utter well being' can be observed when a very young infant is in a state of deep sleep. Absolute tension on the other hand is seen as the maximum possible deviation from absolute euphoria and this can be observed in a state of terror. The interplay between these two forces are such that an individual can

Absolute euphoria and absolute tension

never be either at one end or the other. This suggests that total euphoria or total tension does not exist. Some could be near absolute euphoria, some could be near absolute tension and others could be midway between absolute euphoria and absolute tension.

Tension of needs occurs where there is a disequilibrium in one's being, for example one could suffer a lack of oxygen, water, sugar and adequate body temperature. A state of satisfaction is reached when there is a relaxation of the tensions which are caused by the lack or shortage of these elements. Satisfaction is reached when the infant breathes to compensate for his or her need for oxygen and eats and drinks to remedy his or her need for food and water respectively.

The need for security

The need for security is linked to the tension of anxiety, which according to Sullivan, is induced by the mother and transferred to the infant. This induction of anxiety in the infant can be explained through the concept of what Sullivan called empathy. The implication here is that the infant, through this empathic understanding of the state of his or her mother, experiences anxiety himself or herself. Relaxation of this tension of anxiety will lead to a state of interpersonal security. The need for interpersonal security therefore means getting rid of anxiety. Unlike some of the tensions of needs, the tension of anxiety has no specific sources and the infant is therefore not able to remedy it. 'The infant's capacity for manipulating another person is confined, at the very start, to the manifesting needs, and the person who would respond to manifest need in the situation in which the infant is anxious is relatively incapable of that response because it is the parental anxiety which induces the infant's anxiety' (Sullivan, 1953, p.43).

Ways of dealing with tension of fear

The tension of fear manifested through its most extreme form, that is terror, poses a great danger to the existence of the person. Whilst an infant's way of dealing with the tension of fear is crying, an adult deals with it in one of four ways. These are to:

1   Remove or destroy the fear-provoking circumstances. What people do in this instance is to identify the source of danger and get rid of it.
2   Escape from the situation which is causing the fear. People basically run away from the threatening element.
3   Neutralise the fear-provoking circumstances. If for example a person threatens me with physical violence and I demonstrate to him that I can be as violent as him, the chances are that we will not come to blows.
4   Ignoring the fear-provoking circumstances.

The self system and dynamism

The sense of self or 'self-system' as Sullivan called it, emerges during the first year of life as a result of the interpersonal experiences between the child and the mother. Mother in this context does not necessarily refer to the biological one. This in fact could be almost anyone, man or woman, provided that, that person is the prime carer. The nature and aspect of this interaction and nurturing will dictate the overall impression the child will have of him or herself. Sullivan argued that the child's impression can be any one of the three personifications, and these are Good Me, Bad Me and Not Me.

Good Me

The Good Me emerges as a result of positive experiences from the mother. Sullivan (1953, p.162) explained this as experiences in which satisfaction has been enhanced by rewarding the infant with tenderness because mother is pleased with the way things are going. The implication is that when the mother is happy with the baby, she behaves in a rewarding way towards the latter. The child learns and adopts those behaviours which generate pleasure, happiness and gratification. This reflects one of the sentiments of operant conditioning. The basic premise is, I work out the behaviours which please you and I adopt the same, in return you behave positively towards me. The good me therefore is synonymous with the me which pleases mother.

Bad Me

The Bad Me is induced by a mother who is disapproving of some of the things the infant does. This gives the latter the impression that if mother does not like it, it must be bad and because 'I am doing bad things, I must be bad'. According to Sullivan, the child frequently behaves in a way which causes tenseness on the part of the mother, the latter's response instils the notion of the 'bad me' into the child. Negative feedback from the mother makes the child feel anxious, tense and uncomfortable. The child therefore learns to avoid those behaviours which generate distressing feelings.

Not Me

The Not Me also is induced by the mother through her forbidding gestures and the infant experiences intense anxiety as a result. Sullivan said that the Not Me evolves gradually from a primitive character. This mischievous type of child is received with awe, horror, loathing or dread and disapprovement. In an attempt to rid him/herself of the anxiety that the feelings of awe, horror, loathing and dread bring, the child denies them and concludes that these feelings are not his or hers. This is seen as 'not me'.

Sullivan argued that the developmental history of personality is the developmental history of interpersonal relations. Everything that an individual undergoes or lives through becomes part of his or her experience.

'Experience is the inner component of events in which a living organism participates as such' (Sullivan, 1953, p.26). What one experiences in life is filtered through one's perception of that event. Having said that, it would be wrong to imply that experience is the same as the event in which one is involved in. The implication here is that the act of experiencing is to actually live or go through any event as it occurs. Having experience of the event suggests the act of reflecting on that particular event which one has encountered and by so doing one creates a reality and a link in one's mind between the event and one's present state, that is the state of the here and now. One can therefore assume that reflecting can be both an operant (as in operant conditioning) as well as an automatic or reflexive act (as in classical conditioning). Reflecting can be considered as an operant behaviour when say for example I actively engage myself in looking back at my participation in any event which has taken place in my life, like a holiday or my first day as a lecturer. Reflecting can be regarded as a reflexive or automatic act when my thoughts and or my feelings are unconsciously triggered off by either external or internal stimulus and I re-live that event. Flashback is the easiest example that springs to mind, and it is a case in point to support Sullivan's argument that 'experience is not the same as the event in which the organism participates' (Sullivan, 1953, pp. 26–27).

According to Sullivan there are three modes of experience and these are identified as:

- Prototaxic experience
- Parataxic experience
- Syntaxic experience

Prototaxic experience

Prototaxic experience is described as a primitive kind of experience which is beyond any comprehension and understanding on the part of the infant. The infant deals with what he or she is currently going through and does not make any distinction with either past or future experiences. It is as if I am in a dream and when I wake up, I will only have traces of what the dream was about. This provides me with a rough basis for memory. The emphasis is very much on the here and now. The infant cannot differentiate between self and the rest of the world. This idea is not dissimilar to Carl Rogers' concept of unitary man.

Parataxic experience

Parataxic mode of experience too is momentary and there is no structure to how the child experiences events. Even though some events may occur concurrently, the child is not able to make a logical connection between them. Through group activities however, interpersonal activities and social experience, the child learns the meaning of language in its broadest sense. This experience is described as being more personal and unique to the person who is living through these events. It is also believed that the parataxic mode of experience is frequently the foundation for adult prejudices and superstitious beliefs.

Syntaxic experience

Syntaxic experience is a mode of experience which involves the use of language and symbols in interaction with others. Principles are shared with others and based on a common understanding, these are accepted to be true. According to Sullivan, consensually validated symbols underpin almost everything in the syntaxic mode; what distinguishes syntaxic operations from everything else that goes on in the mind is that they can under appropriate circumstances work quite precisely with other people.

Sullivan believed that when an individual is in transaction with others, he or she tends to adopt numerous strategies which fall mainly into the categories of consensual validation, selective inattention and focal awareness.

Consensual validation

Consensual validation means that an individual measures his or her perceptions with those of others in an attempt to reduce distortions. As Sullivan (1953) said, a consensus would have been reached when the infant has learned precisely the right word for the right situation.

Selective inattention

Selective inattention simply means that one happens not to notice certain things in one's life. The individual ignores or overlooks some anxiety-provoking issues. One, for example, may choose to ignore or deny the existence of a loss.

Focal awareness

Focal awareness suggests that the individual sees or hears what he or she wants to see or hear. I may for example want to hear about my strengths and not about my weaknesses.

Development of personality

Sullivan argued that the survival of an individual is dependent on what he called zones of interaction. These are specific areas or organs of the body, whose functions serve to bring relief of tension to the individual's needs. The implication is that these zones of interaction have a lot to do

Zones of interaction

with a person's experiences. Sullivan used the term 'phenomena of recall and foresight' to explain the dynamics between the zones of interaction and experiences. In principle therefore every experience can be traced back to a particular zone of interaction. Amongst these zones of interaction are the oral, anal, urethral and genital zones. The oral zone goes beyond the mouth and as far as the respiratory apparatus. It also includes the organisation of people's sensory organs, such as sight, touch, gustatory and olfactory.

According to Sullivan personality is developed through a series of distinct stages, and different zones of interaction are involved at different stages. The concept of stages implies the following.

- Each and every individual goes through the same stages in the same order. One would for example start at infancy and work one's way through to adulthood and old age, and in the process one would encounter the eras of childhood, being a juvenile, pre-, early and late adolescence.
- Each stage is organised around a critical or dominant theme.
- Behaviour is characteristically different from one stage to the next.

Infancy

This is the first stage of development and it is from birth to the 'appearance of articulate speech, however uncommunicative or meaningless' (Sullivan, 1953, p.33). The major developmental task of infancy is gratification of needs, the infant's activities are focused around the oral, anal, and urethral zones. For example the infant cries in an attempt to free him or herself from fear, similarly when tension accumulates in the bowel or bladder, the infant would defecate or micturate. This is also the stage where there is an element of total dependence on the mothering person for the relief of his/her needs. The interpersonal need of the child is one of contact.

Childhood

Childhood starts where infancy ends (i.e.) from when the infant is able to formulate sounds of speech and extends to the time when playmates, that is, companions and peers are sought. The child learns to accept that gratification of needs cannot always be instantaneous and is comfortable with delaying gratifying such needs. The child also recognises those behaviours which lead to parental approval. The zones of interaction which are at play include oral, in the form of language, anal and urethral. The child's interpersonal needs include the participation of adults in his or her activities.

Juvenile

This state is identified as lasting through most of the secondary school years to the emergence, because of maturation, of a need for an intimate relation with another person of similar status. This implies the formation of satisfactory relationships with peers. The interpersonal needs emphasise the need for peers and the need to be accepted by others. The elements of competition, compromise and co-operation are defining characteristics.

Pre-adolescence

This has a rather brief chronological time span and ends when puberty starts. From a psychological point of view however, pre-adolescence terminates when the person's sexual interests move from homosexual to heterosexual. The developmental tasks include learning to form satisfactory relationships with people of the same sex. Collaboration, ability to show love and affection, and consensual validation are some defining characteristics. The interpersonal needs include the need for a friend and loved one.

Early adolescence

This is the period of personality development where true genital interest occurs. Sullivan's sentiment reflects the notion that the individual comes to realise the dual purposes of the urethral zone of interaction. As Sullivan (1953) said, the urinary–excretory zone now becomes the more external part of the genital zone as well. The developmental task includes learning to become independent and establishing satisfactory relationships with members of the opposite sex. The need for intimacy is a characteristic feature of interpersonal need.

Late adolescence

During late adolescence, the individual learns to become interdependent. He or she learns to form lasting sexual relationships with the opposite sex. This is also a time when the finishing touches are made to the development of personality. The interpersonal need is that of a heterosexual relationship. The predominant zone of interaction is that of the genital organs.

Adulthood

The individual is now able to enter into a loving relationship with others, where they become as significant as oneself. Although this is not the ultimate goal of life, nevertheless it is seen as the principle source of satisfaction in life. From this stage onward, changes in the individual lead to old age.

Sullivan's theory of interpersonal behaviour suggests that the two prime motivating factors, the need for satisfaction and the need for security, are the main determinants of why an individual behaves the way he or she does. The concept of self is personified in three ways, the good, the bad and the not me, and these are formed as a result of interactions with the mothering person. One's modes of experience develop from prototaxic, parataxic to syntaxic. When people communicate with others they adopt any one of the three strategies, consensual validation, selective inattention and focal awareness. The growth and development of one's personality goes through the stages of infancy through to old age and in the process we encounter childhood, juvenile, pre-, early and late adolescence, and adulthood. These however are dependent on the experiences which occur from our zones of interaction. Our interaction with others remains significant with respect to how we behave.

As far as health care is concerned some of those significant factors which Sullivan's theory highlighted are focal awareness and selective inattention. With focal awareness for example I could choose to hear what I want to hear rather than listen to how it really is. Selective inattention would lead to capturing only part of the true message of what others are trying to convey.

Reference

Sullivan, H.S. (1953). *The Interpersonal Theory of Psychiatry*. New York: Norton.

Psychosocial theory   *10*

Objectives

After reading this chapter you should be able to:

1   List all of Erikson's stages of development
2   Explain the effect of successful resolution of each and every stage on an individual
3   Explain the effect of unsuccessful resolution of each and every stage on an individual
4   Explain the link between Erikson's psychosocial theory and care delivery

Erikson's (1902–1994) psychosocial theory of personality development

Erikson recognised and acknowledged those intrapersonal elements which according to Freud, help to shape a person's personality, he also believed that the significant influences of social forces on personality cannot be ignored. The development of personality occurs in eight stages and these take place over a period of time, which spans from the time a person is born to the time they die. Each of these stages has its own critical period to overcome. Critical periods are those crucial times during an individual's life when specific tasks must be accomplished. The resolution of each of these stages can be either positive or negative. Normal growth and development

Table 10.1
Erikson's (1963) stages of development and the critical tasks to be accomplished

Stages of development	Critical tasks to be accomplished	
Oral–sensory	Basic trust	versus mistrust
Muscular–anal	Autonomy	versus shame, doubt
Locomotor–genital	Initiative	versus guilt
Latency	Industry	versus inferiority
Puberty and adolescence	Identity	versus role confusion
Young adulthood	Intimacy	versus isolation
Adulthood	Generativity	versus stagnation
Maturity	Ego integrity	versus despair

is dependent on the positive resolution of the stages. Erikson (1963) referred to the stages as 'the eight ages of man'. Table 10.1 highlights the stages and their respective critical tasks.

Eight ages of human

Like Sullivan, Erikson believed that there are different body zones which act as interpersonal mediators. The face which includes the oral zone, is the prime mediator. Other body zones include the anal and the genital. From this point of view, there are similarities between Erikson's and Sullivan's thoughts. Furthermore Erikson is described as a Freudian in that he believed in some of the principles of psychoanalytical theory, for example the concept of id, ego, super ego and defence mechanisms. Although there are similarities in their thinking, for example Erikson's first four stages (i.e.) oral–sensory, muscular–anal, locomotor–genital, and latency are similar to that of Freud's first four stages (i.e.) oral, anal, phallic and latency, both these theorists had different ideas about the concept of human development. Whereas Freud concentrated mainly on the irrational id, Erikson focused on the rational ego.

Trust versus mistrust

The oral–sensory stage with the major developmental task of being able to establish basic trust in the mothering person and generalisation of such trust to others

Erikson said that the tell-tale signs of social trust in babies can be detected in the way babies eat, drink, sleep and evacuate their bowels and bladders. For example if babies are at ease and comfortable with these functions, this would suggest trust on their part. Similarly if babies show distress and discomfort during these functions, this would be indicative of mistrust. Other signs are, the willingness of infants to let the mothering person out of their sight without any feeling of distress. This only happens when infants feel that they can rely on their mothers to be predictable in their behaviour. For example if the mother goes out, the infant is certain that she will return. Before reaching this stage however, the infant goes through a state of constantly checking to see if this inner certainty matches the outer predictability. If the infant feels ill at ease during the absence of the mother and this is demonstrated in a display of emotion of unhappiness and suspicious behaviour, this would suggest mistrust on the part of the infant. Mistrust can also be observed in those who display defence mechanisms such as introjection and projection. Both these terms have been discussed in Section I, Chapter 2. In the case of introjection 'we feel and act as if an outer goodness had become an inner certainty. In projection, we experience an inner harm as an outer one. We endow significant people with the evil which actually is in us' (Erikson, 1963, p.240).

The ego's task is to establish basic trust against basic mistrust early on in life. This is based on the quality of the relationship the infant has with the mother. Simply put this suggests, 'it's not what your mother can do for you that counts but the way she does it'. 'Mothers create a sense of trust in their children by that kind of admiration which in its quality combines sensitive care of the baby's individual needs and a firm sense of personal trustworthiness within the trusted framework of their culture's lifestyle. This forms the basis in the child for a sense of personal trust worthiness identity which will later combine a sense of being "all right", of being one-self' (Erikson, 1963, p.241). Erikson's sentiment suggests that parents must show their children that there is a rationale for what they (the parents) are doing.

Autonomy versus shame/doubt

The muscular–anal stage with the major developmental task of being able to gain a sense of autonomy (self-control and independence) within the environment

This stage is seen as the foundation for the individual to experiment and deal with (successfully or unsuccessfully) the conflict of 'holding on' and 'letting go'. Holding on can be both positive and negative. The positive aspect of holding on suggests an element of caring, for example in Erikson's words, to have and to hold. The negative aspect of 'holding on' can be seen in retaining or restraining at all cost. Similarly with 'letting go', from a positive perspective, this suggests, relax and allow the child the freedom to function. Its negative side suggests allowing the destructive forces to reign. Erikson's sentiments point to the role of the environment as being responsible for maintaining the equilibrium between holding on and letting go, where both these concepts are seen as positive. This is the stage for children to establish their own autonomy in whatever they do and the environment should be such that it enhances that process. The environment must also protect the child from the experiences of shame and doubt. The word shame is taken to mean a self-consciousness that others are looking at oneself when one is not ready for it. Phrases like, 'caught with your pants down' and 'to bury your face in your hands', reflect the sentiment of being ashamed. You could, for example, shame me by exposing me when I am least prepared. In children's attempts to be autonomous, if they are looked at in a shameful way, their development and growth would be stunted. As adults, they would seek to exert power over others and 'govern by the letter rather than by spirit' (Erikson, 1963, p.244). When people are ashamed, they can do one of two things, they can try and destroy others or they can wish for their own invisibility. Hence the expressions, 'I could kill you' or 'I wish the ground would open under my feet'. Now imagine those children who are made to feel ashamed and whose behaviour is doubted all the time. As they grow into adulthood, they will be lacking in self-confidence and will doubt their own ability and feel inadequate and incompetent. The successful resolution of this stage is dependent on the supportive relationship the child has with his or her environment.

Initiative versus guilt

The locomotor–genital stage with the major developmental task of being able to develop a sense of initiative free from guilt

As children grow older and stronger, they feel better able to take on greater challenges because of the abundance of energy. Their movements are now more controlled and purposeful. They develop a sense of being able to do things on their own, with a feeling of independence about them. These children are fully equipped with their own initiative to take on new tasks. Initiative in this sense suggests an element of 'doing it my way through my own set of references, for example having explored a situation, I decide on how best to deal with it without help from others. I make it a personal undertaking.' The key issue here is this ability to make decisions on one's own. Erikson (1963, p.84) saw initiative as, 'the selection of goals and perseverance in approaching them'.

Erikson said that infantile genitality plays a crucial role in the task of initiative versus guilt. Guilt results from the fact that although children may contemplate sexual wishes, they have neither the physical ability nor the mental preparation to engage in such activity. This therefore means a block to their initiative. Failure to achieve the end goal brings with it a sense of guilt. This stage calls for an element of self-control of those behaviours which are deemed inappropriate. The danger though, is a possible overreaction on the part of the child, and this can lead to an over punitive kind of behaviour. Children may end up viewing themselves as evil for feeling and thinking the way they do. Resolution of this stage is very much up to the child to achieve. He or she needs to gain insight into the roles and relationships as dictated by society and adapt accordingly.

Industry versus inferiority

The latency stage with the major developmental task of being able to develop a sense of industry (that is to be ready for what is required for later life) without feeling inferior

Successful resolution of the first three stages means that children are now ready to prepare for adult life, that is to work and to provide for others (others is taken to mean those who will be dependent on them, for example children). Realising that they cannot live with their parents forever, they develop a sense of what Erikson called Industry. This means that children learn to adjust to what is required for later life, that is to work and take responsibility to provide for others. Here what is seen as the fundamentals of technology are developed. The danger at this stage is the individual may feel a sense of inadequacy and inferiority. For example if they are not successful in achieving their chosen goals, they may feel disappointed. This may lead to feeling discouraged, they may therefore lose their sense of industry. Erikson said that many times a child's development is disrupted when family does not prepare him/her for school life. This latency stage is one of the most crucial stages in that it involves working with others and demands a sense of collaboration and division of labour.

Successful resolution of this stage sets the scene for establishing a sense of identity.

Identity versus role confusion

The puberty and adolescent stage with the major developmental task of forming a sense of self without being confused as to his or her roles

This stage sees the end of childhood and the emergence of the young person. Physiological changes become more apparent. There is a kind of revolution in the internal dynamics of the young adult. There is a major focus on how they appear to others as compared to how they themselves feel. The quality of experiences in the earlier stages plays a crucial part in that it serves as a foundation which this stage is built upon. This stage sees the young person's search for love. Love also becomes very much the main topic of conversation. Erikson said that this love is these young persons' way of clarifying their own sexual identity. So what they do is to project their own ego-image onto others and by watching their reflections they acquire a clearer picture of their own identities. Other characteristics of this stage are the formation of group cliques and the 'in thing to do' and testing out the meaning of friendship by checking how faithful they are to each other. Negative experiences may induce a sense of confusion in the role the individual takes on and lead to confusion in terms of the individual's sexual identity. Role confusion occurs when the young person's independence is discouraged and significant others may have been authoritarian and puritanical. Role models may have been inconsistent. In such an instance the young person develops a sense of confusion and doubt as to who he or she is.

Intimacy versus isolation

The young adulthood stage with the developmental task of being able to and not being afraid of forming an intimate relationship with another person

Arrival at this stage suggests that these young persons have successfully established their own identities. They are now eager and willing to enter into intimate relationships with others. Intimacy here is taken to include sexual intercourse and closeness in friendships. It could also be taken to mean closeness and commitment to one's work. It is as if these young persons have opened their hearts, to share and commit themselves to others or to their jobs. Young persons are even prepared to endure certain sacrifices in pursuit of this intimacy. If these young persons are able to achieve this task, they will have developed the ability to engage in mutual love and respect for others. If on the other hand the young persons are not able to give themselves to others, they will develop a sense of isolation. Isolation suggests what Erikson called distantation. This means a readiness to isolate themselves and if necessary destroy those people who present a threat to them. This type of behaviour is usually seen in what is described as a loner. Other indications would include those people who are not able to keep a job permanently, and those who cannot show love to others. One can presume here that such a person may have been in a situation where love and companionship were absent during their early developmental stage. In such a case, if you have never had love, you would not know what love is and if you did not know what love was, you would not know how to show it. Interestingly Erikson pointed out that there are partnerships which suggests an isolation *à deux*.

Generativity versus stagnation

The adulthood stage with the developmental task of establishing and guiding the next generation instead of feeling a sense of stagnation

The natural progression from intimacy is to start a family provided that the intimate couple does not engage in isolation *à deux*. Adulthood therefore sees the nurturing of the welfare of future generations. Erikson pointed out that the mere fact of having children does not necessarily mean that a sense of generativity is established. Generativity is indicated when there are true and genuine concerns for the welfare of future generations. In the same sense if a couple is not able to have children, this does not mean that they cannot feel a sense of generativity, such a feeling can be experienced through being productive and creative in other ways, such as in one's job. It becomes clear here how *isolation à deux* can protect a couple from having to face generativity. People who do not achieve a sense of generativity experiences a sense of stagnation, where all they are concerned about are themselves. The picture that springs to mind is self centred and egotistical people who live only for themselves and nobody else.

Ego integrity versus despair

The stage of maturity with the developmental task of reflecting and analysing one's life events, be it positive or negative and deducing a sense of achievement instead of despair

According to Erikson, those people who have cared for things or who have cared for others, can look back with a feeling of contentment of having achieved something in their lives. This is like 'been there and done it' and so when death approaches the individual will not say, 'life is too short' or 'if I can do it all over again, I'll do it differently'. If on the other hand, people conclude from their reflections that they have achieved nothing, a sense of despair would be felt. They would want a second attempt at life.

Psychosocial theory and caring

Erikson's theory emphasises the influence of the environment on growth and development. What can be deduced from this is that basically a supportive environment enhances the successful resolution of the first seven stages. The eighth stage is dependent on self evaluation of the quality of life one has had. Growth and development have, as their starting point, the concept of trust, which serves as a foundation for the other stages. If as a child one discovers trust, then one will not be afraid of the life to come and similarly if as a mature adult one possesses integrity, one will not be afraid to die, if one is afraid to die then one would have achieved nothing. From a psychosocial perspective, the very first conflict which the newborn has to deal with is that of trust versus mistrust. Similarly one could argue that the very first conflict a patient has to overcome is whether or not to trust the carer. A trusting relationship leads to the creation of a psychological environment which is free from undue stress. This task rests with caregivers.

Reference

Erikson, H. (1963). *Childhood and Society*. New York: Norton.

Behavioural and social learning theories 11

Objectives

After reading this chapter you should be able to:

1   Differentiate between the types of learning which behaviourists concern themselves with
2   Explain the concept of classical conditioning and show its link with behaviour in general
3   Explain the concept of operant conditioning and show its link with behaviour in general
4   Describe the basic tenet of social learning theory

J.B. Watson (1878–1958)

Whilst Freud was adamant that the explanation for human behaviour was in the unconscious mental processes, behaviourists believe that the key to understanding people's behaviour rests within the way they react with their environment, the focus being on learned behaviour patterns. Two of the most well known behaviourists are John Watson and B.F. Skinner. Watson came to be known as the founder of behaviourism. Behaviour, according to Watson, can be reduced to a set of reactions to a set of stimuli, given the stimulus therefore, one could predict the reaction and given the reaction, one could state what situation it was that caused the behaviour. Watson's (1930, p.104) conviction in the influence of learning on behaviour was so great that he said, 'Give me a dozen healthy infants, well-formed, and my own specified world to bring them up in, and I'll guarantee to take any one at random and train him to be any type of specialist I might select – doctor, lawyer, artist, merchant-chief, and yes, even beggar-man and thief, regardless of his talents, penchants, tendencies, abilities, vocations, and race of his ancestors.' From Cohen's (1979, p.2) point of view, Watson did more than merely found behaviourism. 'He did much work in a variety of subjects like learning, sex research and child development. He invented behaviour therapy in 1919 though no one else actually did much behaviour therapy till the 1940s.' Watson however, was belatedly recognised for his contribution to the field of psychology. Skinner on the other hand came to be known as the great 'operant conditioner'. The two types of learning which behaviourists concern themselves with are

- classical conditioning/learning and
- operant/instrumental conditioning/learning

Classical conditioning

One could perhaps argue that although the concept of classical conditioning was discovered by Watson, it was Ivan Petrovich Pavlov, a Russian physiologist, who made it popular. The mere mention of classical conditioning leads to such remark like, 'it's Pavlov and his dog isn't it?' The concept of classical conditioning, is based on the belief that anyone can be taught to associate a particular stimulus to a particular response provided the response is reflexive. Pavlov (1927) found that when food was placed in the mouth of a hungry dog, saliva was automatically produced. The dog did not learn to produce saliva, it was an automatic response. Pavlov called this an unconditioned response (UCR). Because food in the dog's mouth caused salivation to occur, food was labelled as the unconditioned stimulus (UCS) (see Figure 11.1).

Food   Saliva

UnConditioned stimulus   Unconditioned response

Figure 11.1
The mere presence of food automatically triggers salivary secretion in the animal

Pavlov discovered that if another stimulus (say a bell) which is neutral to the unconditioned response (saliva) is repeatedly paired with the unconditioned stimulus (which is the food) (Figure 11.2), eventually when the conditioned stimulus (bell) is presented alone, the dog would continue to salivate. This time, because the dog salivated to the sound of the bell, salivation is seen as a conditioned response. This would indicate that the dog has been conditioned to salivate to the sound of the bell alone.

The reason salivation is called an unconditioned response before and during conditioning, is because the dog salivated as a response to the food and not to the bell as such. However, when in the final stage of the experiment (after conditioning has taken place), the bell (conditioned stimulus) was sounded and food did not follow, the dog continued to salivate (see Figure 11.3). Salivation is therefore called a conditioned response.

Classical conditioning can only apply to those behaviours which are reflexive in response. Reflexive suggests that one has no control over such behaviour and some of the behaviours which are exhibited as a result of reflex action include:

- rise in blood pressure
- sneezing
- tears
- coughing
- expressing emotions like fear, disgust, anger and sorrow
- goose pimples
- shivering
- pupillary constriction/dilation to changes in light conditions
- sexual arousal
- butterflies in stomach

- perspiring
- vomiting
- salivation
- reaction to pain
- flinching

Figure 11.2

The first step in the conditioning process. Food is paired with a bell and the animal continues to secrete saliva

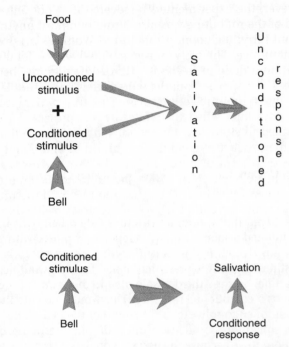

Figure 11.3

Conditioning has been achieved in that the bell alone was able to initiate the secreting of saliva

Stage of acquisition

The acquisition stage of conditioning or learning is the trials during which the dog, in Pavlov's case, learned to make the connection or association between the two stimuli (i.e.) the bell and the food.

Extinction

If the pairing or association of the two stimuli ceases, this will lead to a gradual diminishing and eventual stopping of the conditioned response. The term 'extinction' is given to this phenomenon. If the conditioned stimulus is reinforced with the unconditioned stimulus, then the conditioned response will be strengthened.

Reinforcer

A reinforcer can be described as any event which if it occurs in association with another event will bring about some change in behaviour. For example in the case of Pavlov's experiment, food as the reinforcer brought a change in the dog's behaviour in that it salivated with the sound of the bell. If the reinforcer was to be withdrawn, the dog would carry on responding as if it was still present, but then there will be a gradual decrease in the response, until eventually there will not be any response at all. The concept of reinforcement will be explored further later on in this chapter.

The conditioning of Little Albert

Watson and Rayner (1920) demonstrated how the principles of classical conditioning can be applied to humans in an experiment which involved a little boy and a white rat. The white rat was used to generate fear in the 11-month-old boy who came to be known as Little Albert. Prior to the experiment, Little Albert was not afraid of rats. After conditioning however, the experimenters discovered that not only was Little Albert afraid of the rat but he was also afraid of almost anything which was white and furry, including a rabbit and Watson's mask of a white bearded smiling face. The white rat was paired with a loud noise produced by hitting a gong of steel bar with a claw hammer behind Little Albert's back. The response from the paired stimuli was that Little Albert showed fear by crying and falling over. This trial was repeated seven times and 5 days later when the white rat was presented alone, Little Albert continued to show fear by crying. Watson argued that people's feelings are the product of conditioning and that emotional life grows and develops as a form of habit. Cohen (1979, p.144) wrote, 'Watson had hoped to be able to retrain Little Albert into not being afraid of the white rat. He intended to do this by showing the child the rat far away in the distance while the child felt very secure and slowly building up his tolerance for seeing the rat. But unfortunately Albert was adopted by a family that lived outside Baltimore and so no further tests could be made. Somewhere, perhaps, there is a man of 59 whose name is Albert who maybe has a terror of white rats.' This, one presumes, would have been seen as 'one small price to pay for a giant leap in behavioural research'.

Stimulus generalisation

Watson and Rayner's experiment demonstrated that Little Albert became afraid of all the things which were furry. The answer to this lies in the concept of stimulus generalisation. This basically means that stimuli of similar properties to that of the conditioned stimulus would generate a similar response to that of the conditioned response. Albert was conditioned to be afraid of the little white rat, one of the rat's characteristics was 'furry', so Little Albert became conditioned to most of the things which were furry and the fear of the little white rat became the fear of rabbits, dogs, and fur coats. Although in this instance it turned out to be negative, there are certain advantages to the concept of stimulus generalisation. As Hjelle and Ziegler (1992) said, if this was not the case, then we would have to spend the best part of our lives relearning how to respond appropriately to each situation.

Stimulus discrimination

Stimulus discrimination is the opposite to stimulus generalisation in that in the case of the former, the response is specific to certain stimulus. For example instead of responding to sound in general, I respond to a specific type of sound. In Little Albert's case stimulus discrimination would have meant showing fear only to the little white rat.

Skinner (1904–1990) and his operant conditioning chamber

The implication of classical conditioning is that learning takes place reflexively. Skinner (1953) however believed that this is not sufficient enough an explanation to account for why people behave the way they do. The link is not in what comes before the behaviour, but in the consequences following that behaviour. Operant learning (often known as operant conditioning) is based on the idea that a behaviour is followed by a consequence, and the nature of the consequence influences a person's tendency to repeat or not to repeat similar behaviour in the future. Unlike classical conditioning, operant conditioning is a learned and voluntary response. Emphasis is very much on the nature of the consequences. If the consequence of the response is favourable to the person, then the behaviour is more likely to be repeated in the future. If the consequence of the response is negative, the behaviour is more likely to decrease (see Figure 11.4). For example if I say hello to someone and my hello is acknowledged, I am most likely to repeat this behaviour every time I see that person. If on the other hand my hello is not acknowledged and I am totally ignored, I will probably try one more time and then perhaps stop in my attempt to communicate with that person.

Figure 11.4
Consequences dictate behaviour

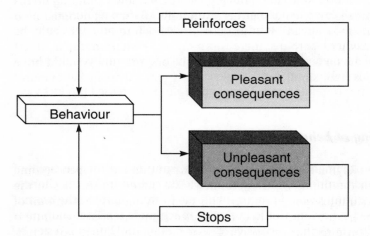

One could argue that the birth of the concept of operant conditioning took place in what Skinner called 'an operant conditioning chamber'. This is basically a box, the dimensions of which left enough room for a chosen animal (this was mainly a rat, a pigeon, or a monkey) to move freely inside. The box is equipped with two mechanical devices: a lever or a key which can be controlled from the inside of the box, and a food dispenser which is controlled from outside the box. A typical experiment would be to place a hungry rat or a pigeon in the box and to reward the animal every time the animal presses on the lever, in the case of the rat (or pecks at the key, in the case of the pigeon). During the early stage of the experiment, it is very much a case of trial and error, but as the experiment goes on, the animal is able to make the connection between its behaviour and the reward. From a behaviourist's point of view, this would prove that the animal is to a large extent responsible for its behaviour, for example the rat will only obtain food if it presses on the lever, therefore the rat learns to press the lever every time it wants the food.

Operant conditioning in humans

The principle of operant conditioning is apparent in most aspects of human behaviour. The reward that one works for ranges from obtaining material things such as money, to receiving love from others. Below are some other examples.

- Bullying. A bully's reward can be anything from personal satisfaction to obtaining material things. So if bullying leads to being rewarded, then the bullying behaviour will persist. If on the other hand the victim stands up to the persecutor, with the message that the latter will not win, the chances are that the bullying will stop. (It must be emphasised here that this is the principle of it, and there is no intention to trivialise the problem of bullying).
- Doing well in an assignment or examination. Here again the scenario is similar. Obtaining good grades will, in principle, spur people to try harder.
- You like someone more if he or she is nice to you and you do not like those who are not nice to you.
- Performance related pay. Managers profit by increased productivity.

The shaping of behaviour

There is an argument to suggest that if one wants to use the principles of operant conditioning to train an animal to do certain tricks, the chances are that the trainer would have a long time to wait. Shaping the animal to the desired behaviour would in fact be much more sensible. Shaping is also called the method of successive approximation and it means a step by step process of reinforcement. If for example you want to train a pigeon to peck at light number 20 in a row of lights, the process of shaping would start by rewarding the pigeon only if it turns in the direction of light number 20. The next stage of the reward would come if the pigeon takes a step forward in that direction and so on. The reward is given on a step by step basis and eventually the animal gets to the target.

Schedules of reinforcement

The concept of reinforcement is crucial to the mechanics of operant conditioning. The frequency and timing of reinforcement or to give it its proper term, schedules of reinforcement, explains why some behaviour will persist long after the reward has been discontinued whilst other behaviour will cease immediately after. During the early stage of any conditioning experiment, the form of reinforcement which is used is called continuous reinforcement. This basically means that every time a desired behaviour is exhibited, the animal or person is rewarded. The disadvantage with this is that it can work out to be expensive and time consuming to maintain the desired behaviour. Furthermore as soon as reinforcement is discontinued the desired behaviour will cease. Most of people's behaviours are reinforced only some of the time. For example a baby will cry numerous times before he or she is given attention. More effective ways of maintaining a desired behaviour is explained through the concept of intermittent or partial reinforcement. There are at least four types of partial reinforcement and these are as follows.

- Fixed-ratio reinforcement schedule (FR). Here a fixed number of responses has to be made before reinforcement (which is predetermined at a set value) is given. For example the rat may have to press the lever 10 times before it will be rewarded. In this case the fixed ratio is 10 to 1, and this suggests that the rat will only be rewarded at every tenth press of the lever.
- Fixed-interval reinforcement schedule (IF). In this instance it is the time interval which is set at a predetermined value and the subject is rewarded at that particular time. For example this could be set at every 5 or 10 minutes, in which case reinforcement is given at every 5 or 10 minutes.
- Variable-ratio reinforcement schedule (VR). The subject is reinforced only after making a certain number of responses and that number varies every time. The subject is therefore unable to predict how often they will be rewarded. A case in point is the one-armed bandit or any other form of gambling machine. The person is left not knowing when he or she will be rewarded.
- Variable-interval reinforcement schedule (VI). The subject is reinforced only after a set time interval but this time interval is different every time. Like the name suggests the time interval varies all the time. Here also, as in the variable-ratio reinforcement schedule, reward is unpredictable.

Primary and secondary reinforcement

There are two types of reinforcement and these are primary and secondary. A primary reinforcer can be described as any event or object that has in itself the properties of being able to reinforce the behaviour. Any reinforcer which does not require prior association with other reinforcers is classed as a primary reinforcer and this includes such things as food, water and sex. This suggests that one does not have to learn that food, water and sex are rewards in themselves. A secondary reinforcer on the other hand needs prior association with other reinforcers to function as a reinforcer. Examples of secondary reinforcers are money and personal achievements like success in jobs. Money on its own is not a reinforcer. Imagine if there was no association between money and basic necessities of life or even life's luxuries, it would be as though it was not worth the paper it is printed on. We use money to buy things. Money on its own does not mean much.

Positive and negative reinforcement

Much of what goes on in life is based on some sort of reinforcement and this can be either positive or negative. A positive reinforcer is any event or object which increases the probability of a response, such as performance related pay, where if one performs well one gets more money. A negative reinforcer on the other hand is any event or object which removes a painful stimulus. If for example a child's screaming is causing me pain, I politely ask the child to stop. If the child stops, then it is most likely that every time the child screams, I would be polite with my request. Similarly if I do not like doing the ironing, this can be used to make me go shopping. Going shopping is the negative reinforcer which prevents the painful job of ironing.

Punishment

Although some people tend to use negative reinforcement and punishment synonymously, nevertheless these are two distinctly different terms. Whereas negative reinforcement encourages a desired response, punishment reduces or terminates the undesired behaviour. An example of punishment would be, your bank charging you £20 for having to write to let you know that you are overdrawn. The probability of being overdrawn again is less than prior to the heavy 'fine'. The same principle is used to deter people from illegal parking.

Social learning theory

The basic tenet of social learning theory is that people learn by observing others. Observation is taken to include watching and listening to others. Past experiences also play a crucial part in that people come to expect that certain behaviour will give them what they want. Bandura (1989) believes that behaviour is mainly regulated by anticipated consequences, and that most of what an individual does is acquired through the influence of watching others. Children pay attention to what adults do and then they repeat what they have seen. Bandura (1969, p.45) argues that the views offered by psychoanalytical theories of personality show behaviour as 'being impelled by powerful internal forces that they not only are unable to control, but whose existence they do not even recognise. On the other hand, behavioural formulations often characterise response patterns as depending on environmental contingencies. The environment is presented as a more or less fixed property that impinges upon individuals and to which their behaviour eventually adapts.' Bandura in fact dismisses both these views as inaccurate and believes that psychological functioning is a continuous reciprocal interaction between behaviour and the conditions that control it. Further discussion on Bandura's ideas is offered in Chapter 7. Similarly the link with self-awareness and clinical practice is discussed in Chapter 8.

References

Bandura, A. (1969). *Principles of Behaviour Modification*. London: Holt, Rinehart and Winston, Inc.

Bandura, A. (1989). 'Human agency in social cognitive theory.' *American Psychologist*, **44**, 1175–1184.

Cohen, D. (1979). *J.B. Watson: The Founder of Behaviourism*. New York: Routledge & Kegan Paul.

Hjelle, L.A. and Ziegler, D.J. (1992). *Personality Theories: Basic Assumptions, Research and Applications*. New York: McGraw-Hill.

Pavlov, I.P. (1927). *Conditioned Reflexes*. New York: Oxford University Press.

Skinner, B.F. (1953). *Science and Human Behaviour*. New York: MacMillan.

Watson, J.B. and Rayner, R. (1920). 'Conditioned emotional reactions.' *Journal of Experimental Psychology*, **3**, 1–14.

Watson, J.B. (1930). *Behaviourism*, revised edn. New York: Norton.

Stress and behaviour 12

Objectives

After reading this chapter you should be able to:

1 Offer at least one definition of stress
2 Explain some of the biological responses to stress
3 Describe Holmes and Rahe's notion of stress
4 Explain Lazarus and Folkman's cognitive appraisal model of stress
5 List and explain Cox's five distinct stages of the transactional model of stress
6 Discuss personality types in relation to the stress concept
7 Explain primary and secondary control
8 Differentiate between internal and external loci of control
9 Differentiate between normal and abnormal anxiety
10 Recognise some of the manifestations of anxiety
11 Explain how a knowledge of stress on the helper's part can enhance health care delivery

Stress concept

There is an abundance of literature on the subject of stress; the focus will therefore be restricted to what will add a different dimension to the concept of interpersonal behaviour. This chapter will begin with a discussion of the stress concept and some of its dynamics and this will include anxiety.

The major problem which stress poses is that of definition. Stress can be viewed as a:

- biological response (Selye, 1976)
- an environmental event (Holmes and Rahe, 1967)
- perceptual phenomenon in the form of cognitive appraisal (Lazarus and Folkman, 1984)
- transaction between an individual and his environment (Cox and Mackay, 1976)

These are just some of the categorisations of stress and its multidimensional nature has meant that one single agreed definition is a virtual impossibility. Researchers and theorists have explored the concept of stress from their own particular preferences. It is pointless to offer a definition of stress at this stage, instead some of the ideas of Selye (1976), Holmes and Rahe (1967), Lazarus and Folkman (1984) and Cox (1978) will be considered.

Hans Selye's biological response model of stress

Selye's (1976) model focuses on the physiological responses of the organism. Selye defines stress as a state which is manifested by a specific syndrome which consists of all the non-specifically induced changes within a biological system. From this perspective the characteristic feature of stress is 'the fight or flight phenomenon'. The way the body reacts to stress is what Selye called 'General Adaptation Syndrome'. This model states that when an organism is faced with a threat, the general biological response occurs in three stages. These are

- alarm reaction
- resistance reaction and
- exhaustion

Alarm reaction

Alarm reaction is the first warning that the organism has about the stressor or stressors. Stressor means anything which carries an element of either physical or psychological danger to the organism. As a response therefore, the organism prepares itself to either fight or flee. Initially the organism experiences a state of shock, after which time, the body prepares itself to deal with the stressor or stressors. The alarm reaction is characterised by:

a   increased blood flow to active muscles and decreased blood flow to organs that are not needed for action
b   increased rates of cellular metabolism
c   increased blood glucose concentration
d   increased muscle strength
e   increased mental activity

Resistance reaction

Resistance reaction is the stage where maximum adaptation occurs. If this is successful then the next stage is avoided. If, on the other hand, the stressor persists at the same or greater intensity and resistance reaction fails, the person then progresses to the third stage.

Exhaustion

Exhaustion has serious implications in that the person has no more energy left to fight against the stressor. This is as though 'I've done everything I possibly can and can't do any more'. In this situation, if outside help is not available, the person may die.

Holmes and Rahe's environmental event model of stress

There is a belief to suggest that certain environmental events which take place in people's life require them to make changes in their established lifestyles. These events can be both positive and negative. Holmes and Rahe (1967) formulated a method of establishing a correlation between life events and illnesses. The tool they developed became known as the Social Readjustment Rating Scale. The scale consists of 43 life events ranging from

Table 12.1
Holmes and Rahe's (1967) life events

Social Readjustment Rating Scale Life Event	Mean value
Death of a spouse	100
Divorce	73
Marital separation	65
Jail term	63
Death of a close family member	63
Personal illness or injury	53
Marriage	50
Fired from work	47
Marital reconciliation	45
Retirement	45
Change in family member's health	44
Pregnancy	40
Sex difficulties	39
Addition to the family	39
Business readjustment	39
Change in financial status	38
Death of a close friend	37
Change to different line of work	36
Change in number of marital arguments	35
Mortgage or loan more than $10 000	31
Foreclosure of mortgage or loan	30
Change in work responsibilities	29
Son or daughter leaving home	29
Trouble with in-laws	29
Outstanding personal achievement	28
Spouse begins or stops work	26
Starting or finishing school	26
Change in living conditions	25
Revision of personal habits	24
Trouble with boss	23
Change in work hours' conditions	20
Change in residence	20
Change in school	20
Change in recreational habits	19
Change in church activities	19
Change in social activities	18
Mortgage or loan less than $10 000	17
Change in sleeping habits	16
Change in number of family gatherings	15
Change in eating habits	15
Vacation	13
Christmas season	12
Minor violation of the law	11

death of a spouse to minor violation of the law. A numerical value is given to each of those events, for example the highest value of 100 is given to death of a spouse and the lowest value of 11 is given to minor violation of the law (see Table 12.1).

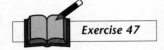

Exercise 47

Have a go at checking out where you are within this scale and highlight those events which are applicable to you. Having done so, add up your total score.

The score can be interpreted as follows:

0–150	Possibility of stress-related illness is insignificant
150–199	You stand a 35 per cent chance of stress-related illness
200–299	You stand a 50 per cent chance of stress-related illness
300 or more	You stand an 80 per cent chance of stress-related illness

Although one could argue that there are various weaknesses to the scale, for example it is rather dated, nevertheless it does offer some indication as to the effect of environmental events on a person's life.

Holmes and Rahe's Social Readjustment Rating Scale does not allow for the fact that some people may score over 300 and yet they may not show any sign of stress-related illnesses. It may well be that these people are well supported or well equipped to deal with the changes in the environment. Having said that it would be true to say that life events are very significant to whether a person stays healthy or becomes ill.

Lazarus and Folkman's cognitive appraisal model of stress

Cognitive appraisal basically means a person's unique self-assessment and evaluation of his dynamic relationship with the environment and how significant that relationship is to him or her. Lazarus and Folkman (1984, p.19) believe, 'psychological stress is a particular relationship between the person and the environment that is appraised by the person as taxing or exceeding his or her resources and endangering his or her well-being'. If for example I perceive that what I am being asked to do is more than I am able to do then my well being is threatened. Although the definition does not take into account the fact that people can suffer from stress as a result of their coping capacities exceeding the demands, nevertheless this has to be recognised as a stress-inducing agent. Hinton (1991) in Spielberger *et al.* (1991) states that both overload (that is where the demands exceed capacities) and underload (capacities exceed demands) can be regarded as causing stress. Stress therefore can be seen as a dynamic process which results from the interplay between appraisal and coping. The emphasis here is not on demand and actual capability but on perceived demand and perceived capability. The role of perception therefore is crucial.

According to Lazarus and Folkman, there are two forms of cognitive appraisal. These are primary and secondary appraisals.

1   Primary appraisal suggests that the person assesses and evaluates
     the environment in order to determine its potential threat. One of
     three conclusions can be drawn from a primary appraisal. These
     are:
     - Irrelevant. This is taken to mean that one comes to the conclu-
       sion that the event or situation bears no significance to the
       lifestyle of the person. As for example saying 'this does not affect
       me'.
     - Benign-positive. This means that it is beneficial to the individ-
       ual. It brings an element of pleasure and enjoyment.
     - Stressful. This implies either harm or loss, threat, and challenge.
       Harm or loss suggests that the person has already experienced
       the damage. This could include a loss, like loss of a job, loss of
       financial security or even loss of a loved one. Threat is related to
       harm or loss except that it has not occurred yet but it is antici-
       pated, like the threat of redundancy, threat of terminal illness
       and so on. The focus of challenge is on the potential for gain or
       growth (see Figure 12.1).

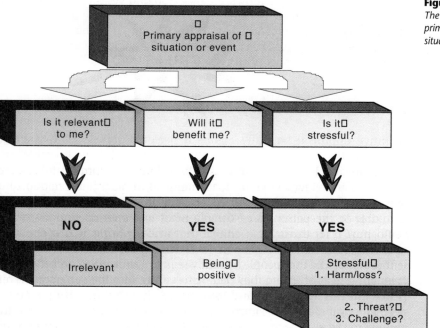

Figure 12.1
*The two possible outcomes of
primary appraisal of a stressful
situation*

2   Secondary appraisal. Here the person assesses and evaluates the sit-
     uation for its potential controllability. For example, 'can I do some-
     thing about the harm or loss, threat, or challenge?' The result of
     this assessment will determine whether the person succumbs to
     stress or not.

Figure 12.2

Shows a secondary appraisal of the situation in terms of its controllability

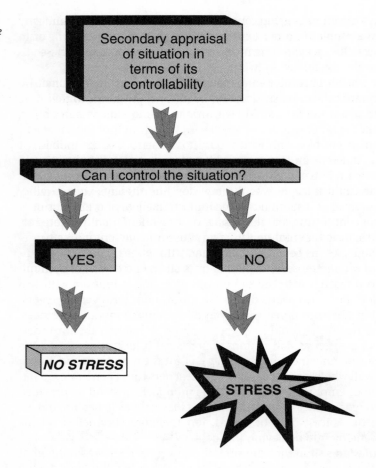

Lazarus and Folkman state that a third kind of appraisal takes place during an individual–environment interaction and this is referred to as reappraisal. Reappraisal is based on new information which becomes available to the person, for example what was seen as benign–positive could now be a threat or a challenge. Similarly what was a challenge could now be a threat.

It could be said that people basically seek to gain control over their environment and in so doing they deal successfully with life's stressors. White (1959) cited in Spielberger and Sarason (1985) stated that people have a need to manipulate and control their surroundings to produce an effective change in the environment. If certain stressors are too challenging or not challenging enough and people are aware of their situation then stress ensues. Although this explanation appears simplistic nevertheless it does demonstrate that perceived ability to cope is crucial to determining whether stress occurs or not. Coping is seen as 'the process through which the individual manages the demands of person–environment relationships that are appraised as stressful and the emotions they generate' (Lazarus and Folkman, 1984, p.19). The demands of person–environment relationships are an interesting concept in that they beg the question, 'why is it that two people may react differently to the same situation?', or to quote Fisher (1984, p.xviii) 'one man's stress may be another man's challenge'. Consider the following two hypothetical scenarios.

James, a teacher in further education, is married with two children. He **Scenario 1** has worked for the same institution for over 20 years, during which time he has had a few confrontations with senior management because he believed that the latter was out of touch with reality, in that management showed no concept of caring with regard to students' welfare. James felt that all his requests were not met and his ideas as to how students could be helped were rejected. He started to show a dislike for his work and at home all he could think of was the raw deal the students were having. James complained of insomnia and feeling extremely tired every morning. He could not concentrate and the quality of his work gradually deteriorated. His physical and mental health gave cause for concern and he subsequently went to see his general practitioner, who referred him to a psychiatrist. James was diagnosed as suffering from stress and a state of burnout.

Jon too is a teacher with the same institution and is married with two **Scenario 2** children. Jon has also worked for the institution for over 20 years. Although Jon does not agree with everything senior management does, nevertheless he felt he could help the students by helping them to raise their level of awareness. Jon as James, perceived a lack of caring on the part of senior management but he believed that the managers had built a solid brick wall which neither students nor teachers could penetrate. So Jon did not even attempt to get through to the managers, instead he provided support and reassurance to the students and his aim was to get into a position where his voice would be heard. Jon therefore channelled all his efforts and energy into achieving this goal.

James' and Jon's situations are similar and yet each showed a different reaction. James was obviously stressed whereas Jon felt challenged. One possible explanation for the differences in behaviour is with the concept of appraisal. From Larazus and Folkman's point of view, both James' and Jon's primary appraisal led them to conclude that a potential stress existed. For James it was interpreted as a threat, Jon saw it as a challenge. During secondary appraisal, James established that the situation he found himself in was threatening and beyond his capability and became ill as a result. Jon's secondary appraisal on the other hand led him to see the situation as a challenge. So he restructured his thoughts and behaviour to take on the challenge. A challenge does not necessarily mean success, it may well be that Jon fails in his venture and in which case the outcome will depend on several other factors, some of which will be explored later on.

Cox's transactional model of stress

Cox (1978, p.18) describes stress as 'part of a complex and dynamic system of transaction between the person and his environment'. There are five distinct stages to this complex system and the starting point is the

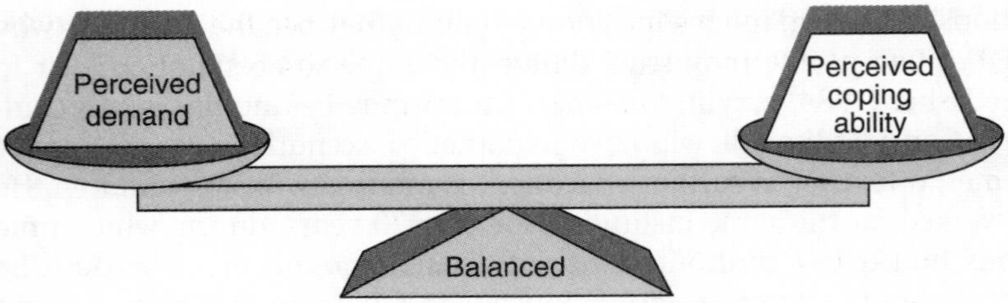

Figure 12.3
A balance between perceived demand and perceived coping ability

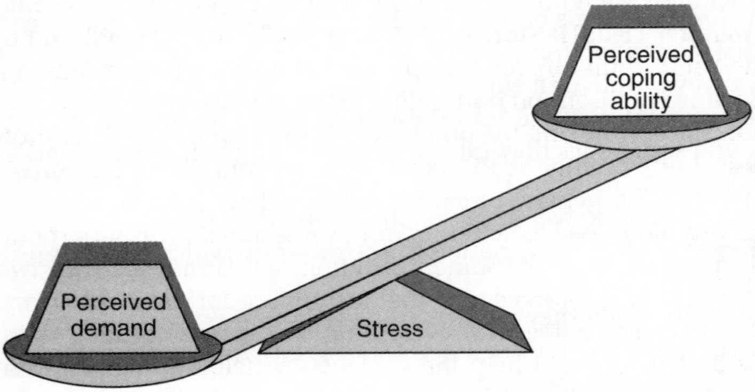

Figure 12.4
A balance between perceived demand and perceived coping ability

demand. Demand is taken to include both internal and external factors. The *second stage* deals with the person's perception of the demand and his ability to deal with it. Stress will be experienced if there is an imbalance between perceived demand and perceived ability to cope.

The key issue at this stage is that of cognitive appraisal, for example if demand is in excess of a people's ability to cope, but the person is not aware of it, they will continue to function as if there is no problem until such a time as they come to realise that they cannot cope. When this happens, stress will ensue. This is like hitting my head against a brick wall without realising that I cannot break through. There is no problem as long as I am unaware of what is happening, but as soon as realisation sets in and I discover that I cannot cope, I become stressed. Could this be why the saying goes something like, 'ignorance is bliss?' The *third stage* is identified as the time when people come to realise that they cannot cope and this in turn initiates physiological changes, followed by cognitive and behavioural attempts to reduce the stressful nature of the demand. The *fourth stage* results from what happens after the attempts to reduce the nature of the demand. The *fifth stage* is feedback and this filters through all other stages.

Common to these perspectives is the issue of coping. It is basically whether people can cope or think they can cope with the demands that make the difference between staying healthy or becoming ill. One particular factor which has some significance as to whether one copes or not is the type of personality one has. Personality is one explanation as to why some people cope whilst others fail to cope. Friedman and Rosenman (1974) used the Type A and Type B personality to identify certain traits and characteristics which are significant in terms of an individual's proneness to illness, more specifically coronary artery disease.

Type A personality

Type A characteristics include:

- A habit of explosively accentuating various key words in ordinary speech even if there is no need for it. They also have a tendency to say the last few words of their sentences far more rapidly than when they first started talking
- Always move, walk and eat rapidly
- Impatient and difficult to restrain from hurrying the speech of others and sometimes they have a tendency to finish other people's sentences for them
- Often attempt to do two or more jobs at the same time
- A tendency to steer conversation in the direction which is of interest to themselves
- Feeling guilty when they attempt to relax
- No longer notice the more interesting or lovely things which they encountered during the day
- Focus on the things worth having rather than on the things worth being
- Set their goal to achieve more in less time
- Feeling challenged, aggressive, hostile towards others who are of Type A
- Exhibit characteristic gestures like clenching fists or banging on the table for emphasis
- Becoming more and more committed to personal activities and the activities of others in terms of numbers

Type B personality

Type B personality includes:

- Being free from all those habits exhibited by Type A personality
- Never impatient and time is not an issue
- No free floating hostility, has no need to impress others unless situation demands
- Playing for fun and relaxation and does not demonstrate achievement at any cost
- Working without agitation and relaxing without feeling guilty

Hardiness of personality

The implication of Friedman and Rosenman's work is that Type A personality is more prone to stress than Type B personality. Kobasa (1979) on the other hand believes that the key to being stressed or not being stressed lies in 'Hardiness of Personality'. A hardy personality is described as a way of managing to remain healthy despite many encounters with stressful situations. The key characteristics of 'hardiness' are:

- commitment
- challenge
- control

Commitment

Commitment is seen as the ability to fully engage in whatever one chooses to do. This could be anything from commitment to one's work, family, society and any other relationships.

Challenge

Challenge means believing that the very existence of life is to be proactive, to search for stimulation, and to experiment.

Control

Control suggests the ability to influence one' own action.

The contrast between 'Hardiness' and 'Non-hardiness' can be seen in Table 12.2.

Table 12.2
Hardy versus non-hardy personality

If people are fully involved in what happens, look at change as a necessity of life and feel in control, then they are less likely to be stressed as compared to those who feel disengaged, threatened and helpless. The latter group is more likely to be stressed.

'Hardiness'	'Non-hardiness'
Commitment	Alienation
Challenge	Threat
Control	Powerlessness

Concept of control

Primary control

Control is as significant as perception in the stress concept. Lazarus and Folkman (1984, p.170) imply that to cope is to control. 'Intuitively it would seem that to cope with a situation is to attempt to control it – whether by altering the environment, changing the meaning of the situation, and/or managing one's emotions and behaviours.' Rothbaum *et al.* (1982) highlight two types of control and these are primary and secondary control.

Primary control suggests an attempt to change the stressful environment. Here the purpose is to make the environment adapt to the person's needs.

Secondary control

Secondary control suggests an attempt to fit in with the environment. Here the person adapts to the needs of the environment.

Locus of control internal versus external

The way people react to stressors is significantly related to how they perceive the element of control. The term 'Locus of Control' is used to refer to the general belief of whether or not an individual's behaviour is under his or her control. Locus of control can be internal or external. An internal locus of control means that I believe I am responsible for what happens to me and an external locus of control means that I believe I am not responsible for what happens to me. As far as dealing with a stressful situation is concerned, those with an internal locus of control are more likely to be confident that they can initiate changes in their environment. Those with an external of control on the other hand tend to believe that they have little power if any to initiate change of any sort. They believe that what happens to them is the result of fate. An internal locus of control therefore can be helpful in reducing stress. Cooper *et al.* (1988, p.56) point out that 'although internal locus of control may help to reduce stress in most situations, they may have even higher stress levels than externals, when presented with a situation over which they actually have no control. Therefore the stress relationship between locus of control and stress responses can greatly depend upon the type of stress encountered.'

The stress concept, although difficult to define, offers a clearer understanding of why some people cope whilst others do not. Many would agree that there are certain common factors which actually dictate why one person may thrive on stress whilst another succumbs to it. These factors include individuality (individuality here refers to the person's own make up), cognitive appraisal of the situation and of one's own ability. A simplistic definition of stress could be 'a perceived or an actual force which works against the organism and under certain conditions leads to ill health'. One such condition could be when stress is persistent and overpowering. In moderate doses stress in the form of arousal can be a performance enhancer, in excess however, it can be a hindrance and leads to ill health. Yerkes and Dodson (1908) showed that the relationships between educational performance and level of arousal conceptualised as fear, is curvilinear (see Figure 12.5).

The argument is that each and every individual needs a certain amount of arousal in order to perform. As the level of arousal increases, so does the performance but only up to its optimum point. If the level of arousal continues beyond the optimum point, then the level of performance would decrease. Yerkes and Dodson's law is widely accepted and can be generalised to almost any dimension of the stress concept. Having said that it is interesting to note the different ways people demonstrate stressful behaviour. Try the following exercise.

Make a list of the ways you deal with a stressful situation.

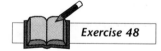

Exercise 48

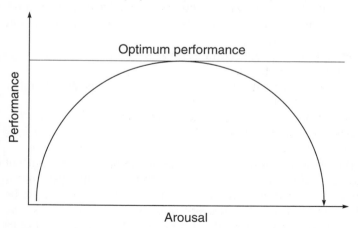

Figure 12.5
'Yerkes and Dodson's curve'. Shows the relationship between level of arousal conceptualised as fear and educational performance as curvilinear. The argument is that performance will rise to the person's optimum as an individual's level of arousal increases, after which point if the level of arousal continues to increase, performance will drop

Broadly speaking the ways one behaves can be categorised under four headings and these are:

1   fight
2   flight

3   freeze and
4   learn and adapt/problem solving approach

If you check your list you will find that it is possible to identify your ways of reacting to a stressful situation under any one or more of the above categories. The first three categories are considered to be maladaptive whereas the fourth one is obviously adaptive. Adaptive is taken to mean the ability to solve problems and to enhance one's growth and development. People can adapt by changing or altering aspects of their environment or they can equip themselves so that they can deal with whatever the stressors are. This suggests an element of 'if you can beat them, you change them, if on the other hand you can't change them, then join them'. Maladaptive behaviours are those defensive behaviours which are exhibited as a response to a stressful event but which do not in the long run deal with the problem.

Fighting my way through, running away from or being petrified with fear cannot be seen as problem solving behaviours but very often are symptoms of anxiety.

Anxiety

Anxiety is a normal emotion as a reaction to fear or apprehension. Everyone has experienced anxiety at some point or other during his or her life. For example people experience symptoms of anxiety when waiting for an interview, getting married or on a first date and so on. Lewis (1977) cited in Sims and Snaith (1988), highlighted six characteristics of anxiety and these are:

1   Anxiety is an emotion associated with the subjective experience of fear or any other related emotions such as terror, horror, alarm, and dread
2   By its very nature, anxiety is an unpleasant emotion
3   Anxiety is focused on the future
4   Either there is no recognisable threat or the threat is generally not in proportion to the level of anxiety
5   The person experiences certain bodily discomfort
6   Bodily disturbances are evident

Normal and abnormal anxiety

Anxiety can be viewed as a reason for the way people behave but not the behaviour itself, for example if I am faced with a fearful object, like a lion, I will not only be anxious but I will also run away. My feeling can be described as anxious, my running away on the other hand cannot be described as anxiety. Sims and Snaith (1988) argue that anxiety explains a person's behaviour, but the behaviour cannot be seen as anxiety. They go on to say that involuntary behaviour such as uncontrollable tremor would be accepted as a direct manifestation of anxiety. The so-called normal anxiety is seen as an emotion which is appropriate to certain situations. If on the other hand the emotion is not appropriate to the situation or that the emotion is out of proportion to the situation, then this would be seen as abnormal anxiety. Abnormal anxiety would be one of those maladaptive behaviours. Anxiety can be either a trait or state. Trait anxiety suggests the anxiety that people carry as part of their personality over a long period of time. State anxiety on the other hand is anxiety which is brought on by a stressful situation over which people feel no control.

Trait and state anxiety

The manifestation of anxiety from a physical perspective can be seen in Table 12.3.

Manifestation of anxiety

Cognitive symptoms include inability to concentrate, irrational think-

Table 12.3
Some of the physical manifestations of anxiety

1	Headaches and migraine
2	Dizziness and light-headedness
3	Blurred vision
4	Facial and other muscular spasms
5	Difficulty breathing
6	Difficulty swallowing
7	Aching at the back of the head
8	Palpitations
9	Angina and chest pain
10	Butterflies in stomach
11	Indigestion
12	Diarrhoea
13	Frequency of micturition
14	Legs feel like jelly
15	Skin rash, like eczema and psoriasis
16	Sweating profusely
17	Sexual difficulties
18	Sleeping difficulties
19	Tiredness

ing, lack of ability to reason, preoccupation, obsession, blocking of words, and pessimistic thoughts.

Affective symptoms include the feeling of guilt, unworthiness, anger, shame and resentment.

Anxiety can be one of the greatest barriers to communication, especially if displayed through aggression. An anxious person comes across as lacking in confidence and is basically incompetent. Carers are role models and as such they are expected to instil confidence in their patients. If they themselves are anxious this will overflow onto their patients, who also become anxious. This scenario is similar to Sullivan's notion that the mothering person induces anxiety in the infant because of the empathic understanding between the latter and his or her mother. The manifestation of anxiety provides some clues as to the effects of anxiety on communication. Anxiety can also be seen as a possible explanation for people's aggressive behaviour.

Anxiety and communication

How the helpers' knowledge of stress can enhance health care delivery

Skilled practice is underpinned by theoretical knowledge, here therefore

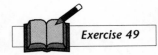

you could try and explain how an understanding of the stress concept can enhance health care delivery.

Below are some ideas to start you off.

- A knowledge of the stress concept would first and foremost enable helpers to recognise and accept their own proneness and vulnerability to stressful influences. By so doing they will be in a better position to protect themselves from a state of burnout.
- Helpers will be able to recognise the relationship between psychological and emotional stress and a physical manifestation. This can enhance the concept of holistic care.
- Helpers' knowledge of stress can facilitate their role as educators of clients/patients. They can advise clients/patients of various adaptive coping strategies. One such strategy may be 'engaging in relaxation exercises'.
- Seyle's biological explanation of the stress concept may enable helpers to recognise clients/patients' physiological reaction to stressors and by so doing may prevent the latter from reaching the exhaustive state.
- Similarly Holmes and Rahe's list of life events can offer some clues as to the effect of accumulation of such events on people's lifestyle.
- Lazarus and Folkman's model focuses on the individual's cognitive appraisal of the event. The model offers helpers an insight into clients'/patients' perception and evaluation of their own situation. This greater awareness can enhance helpers' empathic understanding of their clients.

References

Cooper, C.L., Cooper, R.D. and Eaker, L.H. (1988). *Living with Stress*. London: Penguin Books.

Cox, T. (1978). *Stress*. London: MacMillan Education.

Cox, T. and Mackay, C. (1976). 'A transactional model of occupational stress.' Paper presented to III Promstra Seminar Department of Engineering Production. University of Birmingham, October. Cited in Cox, T. (1978). *Stress*. London: MacMillan Education.

Fisher, S. (1984). *Stress and the Perception of Control*. London, Hillsdale, NJ: Lawrence Earlbaum Associates.

Friedman, M.D. and Rosenman, R. (1974). *Type A Behaviour and Your Heart*. New York: Knopf.

Hinton, J.W. (1991). 'Stress model development and testing by group psychometrics and one-subject psychophysiology.' In: Spielberger, C.D., Sarason, I.G., Strelan, J. and Brebner, J.M.T. (Eds) *Stress and Anxiety*, Vol. 13. London: Hemisphere Publishing Corporation.

Holmes, T.H. and Rahe, R.H. (1967). 'The social readjustment rating scale.' *Journal of Psychosomatic Research*, **11**(2), 213–218.

Kobasa, S.C. (1979). 'Stressful life events, personality and health: an inquiry into hardiness.' *Journal of Personality and Social Psychology*, **37**, 1–11.

Lazarus, R.S. and Folkman, S. (1984). *Stress, Appraisal, and Coping.* New York: Springer.

Lewis, A. (1977). 'Problems presented by the ambiguous word "anxiety" as used in psychopathology.' In: *Later Papers of Sir Aubrey Lewis.* Oxford: Oxford University Press.

Rothbaum, F., Weizs, J.R. and Snyder, S.S. (1982). 'Changing the world and changing the self: A two process model of perceived control.' *Journal of Personality and Social Psychology*, **42**, 5–37.

Selye, H. (1976). *The Stress of Life*, revised edn. New York: McGraw-Hill.

Sims, A. and Snaith, P. (1988). *Anxiety in Clinical Practice.* Chichester: John Wiley and Son.

Spielberger, C.D. and Sarason, I.G. (1985). *Stress and Anxiety*, Vol. 9. Washington, New York, London: Hemisphere Publishing Corporation.

Spielberger, C.D., Sarason, I.G., Strelan, J. and Brebner, J.M.T. (Eds) (1991). *Stress and Anxiety*, Vol. 13. Washington, New York, London: Hemisphere Publishing Corporation.

White, R.W. (1959). 'Motivation reconsidered; the concept of competence.' *Psychological Review*, **66**, 297–333.

Yerkes, R.M. and Dodson, J.D. (1908). 'The relation of strength of stimulus to rapidity of habit formation.' *Journal of Comparative Neurology and Psychology*, **18**, 459–482.

Obedience, conformity, compliance and learned helplessness

13

Objectives

After reading this chapter you should be able to:

1   Define the terms: obedience, conformity and compliance
2   Describe Stanley Milgram's (1974) study on obedience
3   Explain possible rationales as to why people obey
4   Describe Asch's (1952) experiment on conformity
5   Recognise the influence of power and control in relation to obedience, conformity and compliance
6   Define the term learned helplessness
7   Describe Seligman's (1975) experiment on learned helplessness
8   Explain some of the characteristic features of learned helplessness
9   Differentiate between the following attributional styles:
     Internal and external
     Stable and unstable
     Global and specific
10   Explain universal and personal helplessness
11   Explain how a knowledge of concepts such as obedience, conformity, compliance and learned helplessness can enhance care delivery

---

Obedience, conformity, compliance and learned helplessness

'The person who, with inner conviction, loathes stealing, killing, and assault may find himself performing these acts with relative ease when commanded by authority. Behaviour that is unthinkable in an individual who is acting on his own may be executed without hesitation when carried out under orders' (Milgram, 1974, p.xi).

Milgram's concept of obedience focuses on the significant relationship between the environment and the response of the individual. To obey or not to obey, that is not the question, the question is how long before you do as you are told? Obedience, conformity and compliance are all dependent on what is at stake, what people have to lose will dictate to what extent they obey authority. From this point of view, an ordinary person could be turned into a killer, all one has to do to achieve this is to manipulate that person's environment. I could, for example, ask you to kill a total stranger. Your obvious answer would be negative. But then I would tell you that if you do not kill that stranger, I will get the stranger to kill you. You may be altruistic and still refuse, even if you know that the stranger will kill you. I could further manipulate the conditions and threaten the lives of your family or your most intimate partner. Chances are, you will eventually carry out a murderous act. Cruel as this may sound, it does nevertheless demonstrate that almost anyone could be made to obey, even if obeying means killing people. According to Arendt (1963) cited in Atkinson *et al.* (1993, p.762), 'the most ordinary decent person can become a criminal'. The Nazi's extermination of millions of Jews is a grim reminder of the extent to which people will demonstrate their obedience.

Milgram's concept of obedience

Obedience means performing an act under orders from authority figures. This could be anyone from parents to employers. Milgram's (1974) experiment offers some insights into the concept of obedience. The sentiment of the study focused around the issue of 'how far the participant will comply with the experimenter's instructions before refusing to carry out the actions required of him' (Milgram, 1974, p.3).

The basic design of this experiment was to bring two people at a time to a psychology laboratory to take part in a study of memory and learning, at least that was what the subjects were told. The roles of 'teacher' and 'learner' were designated to the subjects. The learner was in fact a confederate, this means that he was acting the role which was scripted for him. The subject being experimented upon was the teacher. The subject was told that the study was about the effects of punishment on learning. The learner (confederate) was seated in the next room, with his arms strapped to the chair and an electrode was attached to his wrist. His instruction was that he was to learn a list of word pairs and whenever he made an error, he would be given an electric shock (the teacher was in fact given a sample shock to enable him to experience the kind of electric shock he was going to administer to the pupil) and the intensity of the shock would increase after each mistake. The shock generator which the learner was connected to had 30 switches, ranging from 15 volts to 450 volts. The sequence of the shocks would start at 15 volts and increase by 15 volts at a time (see Table 13.1).

Table 13.1
A typical example of the voltage of the shock generator

Error	1	2	3	4	5	6	7	→ 30
Volts	15	30	45	60	75	90	105	→ 450

The findings were interesting in that they were beyond what one expected. Try Exercise 50.

Have a guess and make a note of the percentage of subjects you think would go as far as the maximum 450 volts.

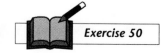 *Exercise 50*

Milgram's findings revealed a staggering 26 out of 40 subjects obeyed the orders to the end. This suggests a 65 per cent total obedience. How far or near were you? When 40 psychiatrists were asked to predict the performance of the subjects, they predicted that only about 0.1 per cent would administer the full 450 volts. In fact a breakdown of the result showed:

- five subjects stopped at 300 volts
- four subjects stopped at 315 volts
- two subjects stopped at 330 volts
- one subject stopped at 345 volts
- one subject stopped at 360 volts
- one subject stopped at 375 volts and
- 26 subjects went all the way to 450 volts

Milgram's study also showed that obedience is significantly influenced by the closeness of the victim. When the victim was in an adjacent room, and out of sight, the result was as shown above. However when the victim was in touch proximity, the result was as follows:

- one subject stopped at 135 volts
- 16 subjects stopped at 150 volts
- three subjects stopped at 180 volts
- one subject stopped at 210 volts
- one subject stopped at 225 volts
- one subject stopped at 255 volts
- one subject stopped at 285 volts
- one subject stopped at 300 volts
- two subjects stopped at 315 volts
- one subject stopped at 345 volts and
- 12 subjects went to the full 450 volts

The overall result showed only 30.0 per cent of the subjects went to the full 450 volts. Perhaps even in obedience there is an element of the 'out of sight out of mind' phenomenon.

Why do we obey?

Why does one obey? The simplest answer would seem to be that one is brought up in an environment where obedience is the norm. No smoking, Keep off the grass, Stay clear, No entry, Don't touch, 30 m.p.h., etc. are all reminders of social rules. Obedience is part and parcel of one's culture. Zimbardo (1992) believes that people obey authority because they want to be liked, accepted, approved by others and they also want to be right.

Hofling *et al.*'s (1966) experiment showed the blind obedience of nurses to the authority of doctors. A group of doctors and nurses investigated whether nurses in 22 different wards of both a public and a private hospital would obey an order that clearly fell outside the boundary of professional practice and hospital policy.

The subject (a nurse) received a call from a doctor who worked at the hospital but whom she had not met. Below is an example of the doctor's conversation with the nurse.

'This is Dr Smith from psychiatry calling. I was asked to see Mr Jones this morning, and I'm going to have to see him again tonight. I'd like him to have some medication by the time I get to the ward. Will you please check your medicine cabinet and see if you have some Astroten. That's Astroten.'

The nurse checked the cabinet and saw the box labelled Astroten 5 mg capsules, usual dose 5 mg, maximum daily dose 10 mg. She then reported that she had found it. The doctor continued,

'Now will you please give Mr Jones a dose of 20 mg of Astroten. I'll be up within 10 minutes. I'll sign the order then, but I'd like the drug to have started taking effect.'

Of the 22 nurses who were the subjects of the experiment, only one nurse refused to administer the drug. The remaining 21 would have easily administered the drug through blind obedience to authority. Although this experiment was conducted some 30 years ago, nevertheless it does demonstrate the impact authority has on the individual.

In general people obey because they have little choice in the matter. For example I will obey if either my life or that of my family is at risk. Similarly an abused person will obey because he or she has no choice. Furthermore the fear of the consequences of disobedience may be too traumatic to even think of.

Make a list of some of the situations where you have obeyed authority. Reflect on what was at stake and what would have happened if you hadn't obeyed.

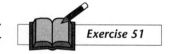

Exercise 51

Conformity

Conformity is another one of those concepts which suggests that an individual's behaviour is clearly influenced by others. Bass (1960) defined conformity as a behaviour which reflects the successful influence of other persons. There is an element here of behaving according to group pressure. When group pressure forces an individual to give in under either the promise of a reward or the threat of rejection, this is called normative conformity. When an individual behaves as others do in order not to appear foolish or inexperienced, this is referred to as informal conformity. This type of conformity can be associated with Asch's (1952) experiment, where subjects were asked to participate in a study which involved visual perception. The subjects were shown cards with three lines of different lengths (Comparison lines). They were then shown another card which had one line (Standard line). One of the comparison lines would be the same length as the standard line. Subjects were asked to indicate which of the comparison lines was the same length as the standard line (see Figure 13.1).

Normative conformity

Informal conformity

Figure 13.1
A typical example of Asch's experiment on conformity

B

aod   1

The experiment would involve anything from seven to nine subjects and only one of the subjects would be the genuine subject. The remainder would be confederates (actors). The confederates acted according to the script. The experimenter would ask each subject to match the lines. The seating arrangement was such that the genuine subject would be the last (or near to last) to give his answer. On the first three trials everyone gave the correct answer. On the fourth trial, the first person gave the wrong answer and so did the second, third, fourth and so on until it was the genuine subject's turn. The genuine subject had realised that the others were wrong but he had to decide whether to go along with the others or act independently. Different studies were carried in the research programme and the findings were as follows:

• 25 per cent of the subjects remained completely independent
• between 50 and 80 per cent of the subjects conformed with the false majority

Asch's (1952) explanation of the rationale for the conformity is that people feel the need not to appear different to the majority in these situations. This phenomenon explains why when students are asked to give feedback on how they feel the session went, there is a tendency to go with what the first few students have said. Zimbardo (1992) explains that a person is more likely to conform when:

• a judgement task is difficult or ambiguous
• the group gels together well and the individual feels attracted to it
• the members are seen as competent and the person feels relatively incompetent on the job
• the person's responses are made public

Ingrational conformity

The one other type of conformity is called ingrational conformity and this suggests that the individual behaves as others in an attempt to be accepted or to impress.

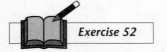
Exercise 52

Make a list of the different situations where your behaviour may have had elements of conformity. If possible identify the types of conformity involved.

Compliance

Compliance reflects any behaviour exhibited as a response to a direct request or wish of an influencing source. Kelman and Hamilton (1989, p.104), state that compliance occurs when 'an individual accepts influence from another person or a group in the hope of achieving a favourable reaction, or avoiding an unfavourable reaction, from the other'. Personal observation suggests that students who are new to a course are more compliant than other groups of students and the same goes for newly-admitted patients. This may be because of their need for acceptance and security. One may behave according to expectation, not because one likes to do so, but because one feels it will have the desired social effect. Compliance is very much part of an individual's interpersonal behaviour and can be seen as a way of life. It would be true to say that perhaps everyone, at one point or another, has complied to a certain situation. People do so at home, in school, at work and various other places. Like obedience and conformity, although people behave according to a set of rules, they retain their true beliefs and their thoughts are not altered. The scenario is completely different with the two other processes of social influence, which are identification and internalisation. Identification is one of the mental defence mechanisms and here it suggests that 'an individual adopts a behaviour associated with a satisfying self-defining relationship to another person or a group' (Kelman and Hamilton, 1989, p.104). In this case there is a change of beliefs, the individual in fact changes his or her beliefs and takes on the beliefs of the role model. Internalisation is believed to occur when an individual 'accepts influence because the induced behaviour is congruent with his value system' (Kelman and Hamilton, 1989, p.107). *Identification*

Internalisation

There are at least four ways of influencing the extent to which an individual will comply to a request and these are:

1 Lowered self-esteem. Aspler (1975) suggests that if people are made to appear foolish in front of others, the chances are that they will comply easily because they want to recover loss of face.
2 Reciprocation. Regan's (1971) study shows that if you have done me a favour in the past, then I am most likely to comply to your request.
3 Foot in the door. If a small request is made first, then when a larger request follows, people comply easily to the larger request. The reverse is also true.
4 Transgressions. According to Wallace and Sadella (1966), if people are caught red handed, in doing something that they should not have done, they are more likely to comply. This is not dissimilar to the concept of 'cash for questioning' where a member of parliament allegedly accepts a sum of money (from someone who will benefit in one way or another) for asking a question in the House of Commons.

The whole issue of obedience, conformity and compliance emphasises power and control. The person who wields the rod of power dictates the extent to which one obeys, conforms or complies. This is clearly illustrated in Zimbardo's (1992) concept of deindividuation. 'On a summer Sunday in California, a siren shattered the serenity of college student Tommy Whitlow's morning. A police car screeched to a halt in front of his home. Within minutes Tommy was charged with a felony, informed of his constitutional rights, frisked, and handcuffed. After he was booked and fingerprinted, Tommy was blindfolded and transported to the Stanford County Prison, where he was stripped, sprayed with disinfectant, and issued a smock-type uniform with an I.D. number on the front and back. Tommy became Prisoner 647. Nine other college students were also arrested and assigned numbers. The prison guards were not identified by name, and their anonymity was enhanced by khaki uniforms and reflector sun glasses' (Zimbardo, 1992, p.575). The prisoners never saw the guards' eyes and were each referred to as 'Mr Correctional Officer, Sir'. At the time of the experiment neither Tommy, nor any of the other nine prisoners knew that they were subjects in a prison experiment. Both prisoners and guards were in fact college students, who had answered a newspaper advertisement and agreed to be the subjects in a 2-week experiment on prison life. Zimbardo (1992) says that everyone in the prison, guards and prisoners were selected from a large pool of student volunteers who had been judged as law abiding, emotionally stable, physically healthy, and what could be described as normal-average. The assigned roles were randomly selected by the flip of a coin. In roles, the guards became extremely cruel and sadistic, the prisoners were passive and helpless. The guards would deliberately manipulate environmental conditions to ensure total obedience. For example failure to obey would lead to the loss of privileges. On occasions prisoners were made to wash toilets with their bare hands, 'doing push-ups while a guard stepped on the prisoner's back, and spending hours in solitary confinement. The guards were always devising new tricks to make the prisoner feel worthless' (Zimbardo, 1992, p.575). This 2-week experiment had to be prematurely terminated after only 6 days because of the extreme stress reaction showed by the prisoners. Zimbardo believes that one should never underestimate the power of a bad situation to overwhelm the personalities and good upbringing of people.

Learned helplessness and dependency

Zimbardo's notion of deindividuation shows how loss of one's identity leads to total obedience to authority. Milgram's concept of obedience suggests the importance of environmental influences on behaviour. Seligman's (1975) concept of learned helplessness shows how cognitive appraisal of the environment influences one's behaviour. In this instance it is one's perception of the situation which causes the pain and not the situation itself. The enemy is within oneself and it is as if one becomes a prisoner of one's own thoughts.

Uncontrollability

Seligman defined helplessness as a psychological state that frequently results when events are uncontrollable. The key word in this definition is 'uncontrollable,' and would suggest that an organism is not able to do anything to influence the outcome of an event. There is an element of a predetermined consequence, that is, whatever one does, the result will be the same. This is just like a no win situation, 'heads I win, tails you lose.' The term 'learned helplessness' is applicable to any situation where an organism has experienced trauma (this means a bad or negative experience) it cannot control and fails to respond in order to avoid future trauma. The root of the concept of learned helplessness can be traced as far back as 1948, when Mowrer and Viek, according to Gilbert (1992), found that if rats were pre-treated with inescapable shock they demonstrated subsequent deficits in escape avoidance learning. Seligman (1975) stated that learned helplessness was discovered quite by accident, whilst working with his colleagues, Maier and Overmaier, in 1967. At that time they were studying the effects of inescapable shock on escape-avoidance learning in dogs. They found that dogs first given Pavlovian conditioning with inescapable shock became profoundly passive later on when they were given escapable shock. The procedure would involve strapping a dog into a hammock and inducing between 60- to 85-second inescapable shocks. The shocks are described as moderately painful, but not physically damaging. During this, the first stage of the experiment, whatever the dog did, it was not able to escape the shock. After a time interval of 24 hours had elapsed, the dog was then placed in a two-compartment shuttlebox. In contrast to the hammock, it was possible for the dog to escape shock in the shuttlebox and to achieve this all the dog had to do was to jump back and forth across the barrier. Seligman and his colleagues found that after the period of inescapable shock in the hammock, when placed in the shuttlebox and when the shock was turned on, the dog moved about frantically for about 30 seconds then laid down and accepted the shock passively. The period of inescapable shock in the hammock would seem to have 'sapped' the dog's motivation to produce any kind of response to avoid the shock. Seligman concluded that the dog had learned to be helpless.

The validity of Seligman's conclusion rests with a comparison study of two other groups of dogs. In the first group the dog received escapable shock whilst in the hammock and in the second group the dog received no *Motivational deficits* shock at all. In the second stage of the experiment both dogs readily jumped back and forth in the shuttlebox thus avoiding the shock. Seligman (1975, p.22) concluded that the shock itself does not produce helplessness, instead it is the uncontrollability of the shock that produces the motivational deficits. 'When an organism has experienced trauma it cannot control, its motivation to respond in the face of later trauma wanes.' Another aspect where the helpless dog was found to be deficient *Cognitive deficits* was that, even if the dog made a successful escape from the shock, it was not able to capitalise on this and failed to repeat it on subsequent trials. That is, after a successful escape, the dog would revert back to the passive behaviour of just lying in the shuttlebox, in contrast to the other groups of dogs that were quick to repeat the successful response.

A further feature of the outcome of learned helplessness is that there is *Emotional disturbance* emotional disturbance. To support this, Seligman (1975) points to the evidence that exposure to uncontrollable trauma produced more conditional fears, ulcer, weight loss and defecation in animals than controllable shock. The belief is that trauma produces emotional disturbances in both animals and humans. Seligman found that there is a time course of learned helplessness in '. . dogs, and that is if the dog is placed in the shuttlebox within 24 hours after uncontrollable shock in the harness, it will be helpless, on the other hand if the interval is 72 hours or longer, the dog will show escapable behaviour'. This would seem to indicate that 'one experience with uncontrollable trauma produces an effect that dissipates in time' (Seligman, 1975, p.41). The above discovery on its own does not show how emotional disturbance is displayed, however if compared to 'disaster syndrome' in humans, the picture becomes clearer. For example when people are actually involved in a disaster, say, a tornado, they function very well, 'but soon thereafter, the victims become nearly stuperous for about 20 hours. After another day or so, people begin to pick up the pieces and go about their business' (Seligman, 1975, p.40).

So far Seligman's theory of learned helplessness is quite strong in terms of animal behaviour, the question therefore is, where do humans fit into this theory? Seligman believes that learned helplessness exists in humans as well. A triadic design (triadic design basically means a design which involves three sample groups, for example in this case group 1 can be escapable, group 2 can be inescapable and group 3 no shock) similar to that of the dog experiment was used with non-depressed volunteers, the electric shock was replaced by noise (escapable, inescapable and no noise). The results were found to parallel those of the animals. The three components of motivation, cognition and emotion are all affected in a negative manner when both animals and human beings are in learned helplessness situations. Seligman argues that the basic cause of all these deficits are due to the fact that both the animal and human come to learn that responding will be futile. Whilst it would be difficult to know the mechanics behind learned helplessness in animals, Seligman and his colleagues (Abramson et al, 1978) considered the concept of attribution as a way of explaining what actually causes humans to be helpless. The attribution style associated with learned helplessness can be considered from three dimensions and these are internal versus external, stable versus unstable and global versus specific.

Internal versus external attributional style

The internal versus external attribution can be explained in terms of how the person perceives the situation. If faced with an unsolvable solution or puzzle, a person believes that he or she is not clever enough to solve the problem, then the explanation for failure is classed as internal. If on the other hand the person believes that the problem itself is unsolvable, then this is attributed to external factors. Seligman (1975) argues that attributing failure to solve problems to internal factors leads to lowered self-esteem, whereas attributing failure to external factors does not. Dweck (1975) studied a group of 12 children to determine whether altering attributions for failure would enable learned helplessness children to deal more effectively with failure and concluded that the children most likely to give up in the face of failure took less personal responsibility for successes

Time is 'a healer'

Stable versus unstable attributional style

and failures and tended to attribute the outcomes of their behaviour to ability rather than effort. Helpless children therefore see themselves as less instrumental in determining outcome, or to put it simply, their locus of control is external.

Failure to solve problems because one is not clever enough would suggest an element of permanency. 'I am not clever enough, therefore I will never be able to solve the problem.' The attribution style therefore is stable as compared to unstable when not being able to solve the problem is associated with say lack of preparation or not feeling well on the day. Seligman argues that if attributional style is stable then the deficit will be permanent, if on the other hand the cause is unstable, failure is seen as temporary.

Global versus specific attributional style

Failure can be considered in terms of its generality and specificity, for example 'I am unable to do this task therefore I am useless'. The implication here is that 'I will not be able to do anything else because I am useless'. The attributional style is described as global, which suggests that failure could result in a wide variety of situations. In contrast to specific problems, when the person believes that he or she is not equipped to deal with this particular problem but given the right conditions and environment he or she may be successful with other problems.

Seligman *et al.* (1979) carried out a study on depressed and non-depressed college students and found that the depressed students attributed bad outcomes to internal, stable and global causes. Furthermore good outcomes were associated with external and unstable causes. Gilbert (1992) pointed out that Seligman's learned helplessness theory and Beck's (1967) cognitive theory of depression made opposite predictions about self-attribution, for example Beck saw people with depression tending to blame themselves for negative outcomes. This would be an internal attribution. In learned helplessness, negative outcomes are themselves seen as uncontrollable. This is an external attribution. Learned helplessness theory therefore was reformulated to agree with Beck's theory. Abramson *et al.* (1980) propose two types of helplessness and these are universal helplessness and personal helplessness.

Universal helplessness

Universal helplessness suggests that an individual has the belief that neither he or she nor anyone else can do anything about the situation. This is demonstrated in diseases like leukaemia, AIDS, cancer and other terminal conditions. If for example I develop a terminal form of cancer, I will come to believe that there is nothing I can do about it. Similarly if you have the same type of cancer, you too will not be able to do anything about it. This implies that both you and I are in the same boat.

Personal helplessness

Personal helplessness on the other hand suggests that an individual believes that he or she cannot control the situation but others may well be able to do so. For example I may come to believe that I am not clever enough to pass my psychology assignment, but others can do so without any problem.

It could be argued that in many ways one is consciously or unconsciously taught to be helpless. Try Exercise 53.

Exercise 53

Make a note of all those behaviours which could suggest an element of learned helplessness.

My list of behaviour would include any behaviour where there is some dependency, for example if I do things for you all the time then you come to learn to depend on me.

Husband depends on wife or wife depends on husband
Patients depend on drugs/alcohol
Patients depend on helpers/carers
Patients depend on hospitals

Dependency and caring

The whole mechanism of dependency can be explained through Berne's concept of symbiosis, where two people share one set of ego states (see Figure 13.2).

Figure 13.2
Two people share one set of ego states

Conditi

Bell

In this case both people are dependent on each other and cannot function as two whole persons separately, but together, they are one. One is helpless without the other and vice versa. This type of relationship is sometimes seen in marriages, where a couple have intimate relationships with one another. Here the relationship is taken beyond Erikson's concept of intimacy, where a person is able to fuse his or her identity with someone else's without fear of losing something of his or her own. Erikson saw this aspect of intimacy as essential for establishing a meaningful marriage. This intimacy however can be a problem if one or both partners lose their identity in the process and become over-dependent on the other. A possible learned helplessness scenario is created and the couple could function as if they were one person (see Figure 13.3).

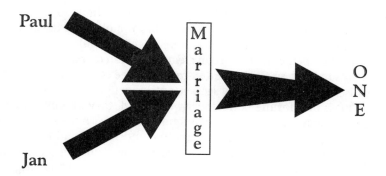

Figure 13.3
Paul and Jan's identities have merged and the dominant one assumes control and responsibility

Figure 13.3 shows the fusion of Paul and Jan's identity in a marriage and the end-product is that the dominant personality will assume the overall identity. For the sake of argument, let us say that Paul is dominant. Therefore Jan's situation will be akin to her being on a tandem and not pedalling. All the pedalling is being done by Paul. If Paul and Jan should split up, Jan would end up helpless because she would not have a clue what to do. Figure 13.4 shows the same couple but with a different scenario. This time both identities (although closer to each other) remain separate. A split between Paul and Jan will leave the latter independent.

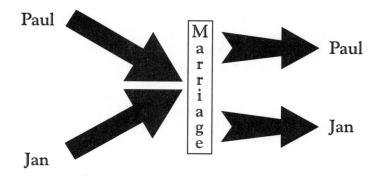

Figure 13.4
Paul and Jan, although intimate, have managed to retain their separate identities and function as two independent people

The relationship between a patient and a helper can in fact follow a similar pattern of behaviour to that of Paul and Jan. If the patient adopts the role of being a passive recipient of care and the helper encourages such behaviour, the patient will end up being dependent on the former, and therefore will not be able to grow and develop as an autonomous being. Here again the helper's self-awareness will determine the future course of action.

There are some fundamental questions which one can ask as far as patients' obedience is concerned.

Helper's knowledge of these concepts can influence health care delivery

* Why do patients obey?
* Do they have any choice?

On the face of it one could say 'no, patients do not have to obey,' but if your life was in someone else's hands wouldn't you obey? This is one of the dilemmas which many patients face. Here it seems a matter of not having any choice. The helper therefore can create a less threatening environment for patients to be in so that the latter may feel free to self express. Helpers of any discipline are commonly seen as authority figures, for example 'we know what is best for the patients'. On their part, they blindly trust us to help them to grow, develop and be autonomous. One's knowledge of these concepts would create more of an empathic understanding towards these patients. It needs to be recognised and accepted that obedience, conformity and compliance are not altogether negative. Sometimes adopting these behaviours can actually save lives, for example, following doctor's instruction and taking one's medication. The helper can in fact support other disciplines in gaining the patient's compliance with treatment. One can conclude, from what Zimbardo (1992) has said, that patients too will comply because they want to be accepted. This is in fact Stockwell's (see Chapter 8) sentiment in her concept of the 'unpopular patient'. The carer therefore needs to be able to offer help unconditionally, as in Rogers' (1951) concept of unconditional positive regards. As a résumé therefore the helper could focus on the following in his/her attempt to enhance health care delivery.

- Inform them about their choices
- Offer options
- Encourage autonomous behaviour
- Offer a supportive environment
- Encourage individuality (this will reduce the Asch effect)
- Treat them with respect and warmth
- Be genuine in your approach
- Enhance self-esteem (see Aspler, 1975, p.188)
- Self-awareness (this will prevent unconscious incompetence)
- Look at patients beyond their role (human being)

References

Abramson, J.Y., Seligman, M.E.P. and Teasdale, J. (1978). 'Learned helplessness in humans: Critique and reformulation.' *Journal of Abnormal Psychology*, **87**, 49–74.

Abramson, L.Y., Garber, J. and Seligman, M.E.P. (1980). 'Learned helplessness in humans: An attributional analysis.' In: Garber, J. and Seligman, M.E.P. (Eds) *Human Helplessness. Theory and Applications*. New York, London, Toronto, Sydney, San Francisco: Academic Press.

Arendt, H. (1963). *Eichman in Jerusalem: A Report on the Banality of Evil*. New York: Viking Press. Cited in Atkinson, R.L., Atkinson, R.C., Smith, E.E. and Bem, D.J. (1993). *Introduction to Psychology*, 11th edn. London: Harcourt Brace College Publishers.

Asch, S.E. (1952). *Social Psychology*. Englewood Cliffs, NJ: Prentice-Hall.

Aspler, R. (1975). 'Effects of embarrassment on behaviour towards others.' *Journal of Personality and Social Psychology*, **32**, 145–153.

Atkinson, R.L., Atkinson, R.C., Smith, E.E. and Bem, D.J. (1993). *Introduction to Psychology*, 11th edn. London: Harcourt Brace College Publishers.

Bass, B.M. (1960). *Leadership, Psychology, and Organisational Behaviour*. New York: Harper and Row.

Beck, A.T. (1967). *Depression: Clinical, Experimental, and Theoretical Aspects*. New York: Harper and Row.

Dweck, C. (1975). 'The role of expectation and attributions in the alleviation of learned helplessness.' *Journal of Personality and Social Psychology*, **31**(4), 674–685.

Gilbert, P. (1992). *Depression. The Evolution of Powerlessness*. London: Lawrence Earlbaum Associates.

Hofling, C.K., Brotzman, E., Dalrymple, S., Greaves, N. and Pierce, C.M. (1966). 'An experimental study in nurse–physician relationships.' *Journal of Nervous and Mental Disease*, **143**, 171–180.

Kelman, H.C. and Hamilton, V.L. (1989). *Crimes of Obedience: Toward a Social Psychology of Authority and Responsibility*. New Haven and London: Yale University Press.

Milgram, S. (1974). *Obedience to Authority: An Experimental View*. London: Tavistock.

Mowrer, O.H. and Viek, P. (1948). 'An experiment analogue of fear from a sense of helplessness.' *Journal of Abnormal Psychology*, **43**, 193–200.

Regan, D.T. (1971). 'The effects of a favour and liking on compliance.' *Journal of Experimental Social Psychology*, **7**, 627–639.

Rogers, C.R. (1951). *Client Centred Therapy*. London: Constable.

Seligman, M.E.P. (1975). *Helplessness*. San Francisco: W.H. Freeman.

Seligman, M.E.P., Abramson, L.Y., Semmel, A. and Baeyer, C.V. (1979). 'Depressive attributional style.' *Journal of Abnormal Psychology*, **88**(3), 242–247.

Wallace, J. and Sadella, E. (1966). 'Behavioural consequences of transgression: The effects of social recognition.' *Journal of Experimental Research and Personality*, **1**, 187–194.

Zimbardo, P. (1992). *Psychology of Life*. London: Harper Collins.

Group dynamics, leadership, and communication

14

Objectives

After reading this chapter you should be able to:

1 Identify some of the criteria by which a group can be defined
2 Recognise the various groups you belong to
3 Explain what group dynamic is
4 Describe Schutz's (1958), Tuckman's (1965), Yalom's (1985), and Bion's (1961) notions of group development
5 Explain some of the factors which can influence group behaviour
6 Define role and describe its four criteria
7 Describe some of the roles within groups
8 Define leadership and explain its different styles
9 Explain some of the facets of leadership
10 Identify the different communication networks within any group

Groups

A group can be described as two or more people interacting with one another in such a way that each person influences and is in turn influenced by the other. According to Baron and Byrne (1991, p.437), a group 'consists of two or more interacting persons who share common goals, have a stable relationship, are somehow interdependent, and perceive that they are in fact part of a group'. This particular definition is taken beyond the 'gathering of a number of people', for example one cannot call two or more people in a shop, a group. There needs to be a certain criteria which dictates what constitutes a group and in fact Baron and Byrne have highlighted such a set of criteria which they argue, needs to be met by any assembly of people for the label of group to be applicable. These are:

1 Interact. This suggests that the members should interact with one another.
2 Interdependent. The implication is that what happens to one member will influence the behaviour of the other members.
3 Stable. The relationship must last for a significant length of time, this could be weeks, months or years.

4   Shared goals. Here at least some goals must be common to all members.
5   Structure. The function of each member must have some sort of structure in that they all have a set role.
6   Perception. Members must perceive themselves as being part of the group.

Group dynamics

Group dynamic is a process which indicates that changes take place at both personal and group level. At a personal level changes may be that of attitude, and a general way of behaving. From a group level this could include roles, relationships, morale and leadership.

Identify the various groups you belong to and check if the above criteria are applicable, for example do you share the same goals? Do you perceive yourself as part of the group?

Exercise 54

Numerous groups can be identified which would fit in those criteria. For example an action learning group may have all the above criteria. Having said that if one or two of those criteria are missing, it could still be called a group.

Group development

Sometimes the goals of the group will determine its membership and its group life. Group life suggests the overall emotional development of any particular group.

Schutz's (1958) FIRO (Fundamental Interpersonal Relations Orientation) theory of interpersonal behaviour suggests that people behave according to their orientation to other people and this is based on three fundamental needs of every group member. These needs are   ***Schutz's perspective***

*   inclusion
*   control and
*   affection

Inclusion is taken to mean the 'area of human contact' Schutz (in Blumberg *et al.*, 1983, p.479). The decision of 'am I in or am I out' is contemplated. Schutz states that human preferences for inclusion vary from oversocial, which is where people feel anxious when they are on their own, to undersocial, where they feel anxious when in the company of others. The need for togetherness is reflected in the way people behave, for example they behave in a way to attract the attention and interest of other members of society.   ***Inclusion, the in–out dimension***

Control is the area of power and influence. Human preferences vary from autocratic, which Schutz sees as a condition where people feel anxious   ***Control, the top–bottom*** when they are not in control, to abdicratic, where they feel anxious when they are in control. People who have a high need for control may display rebellious behaviour and may show their refusal to be controlled. Those with a high need to be controlled may show compliance and submissiveness.

Affection, the near–far dimension

Affection is the area of intimacy with one other member of the group. Human preferences vary from overpersonal, which is where members feel anxious when they are not dealing intimately with other members of the group, to underpersonal, with anxious feeling when they get close to other group members. Those persons with a high need for affection will be friendly, whereas others may avoid closeness and intimacy.

According to Schutz, the development of any group, whatever its size, has inclusion, control and affection as its basic structure. 'Group members separate from each other by going through these phases in the opposite order' (Schutz, 1983, p.479). Group development is also dependent on group compatibility, and this suggests the need for a high degree of reciprocal role preference, for example if I am a person who wants control, then I need to be with someone who wants to be controlled. Similarly if I like to be controlled, then I will feel the need to be with someone who will offer me that element of control.

Group formation

Groups are formed for different reasons, for example to work, learn, and to play. You will have deduced from Exercise 54 that you yourself are a member of various groups and you have your own particular reasons as to why you have joined your groups. According to Tuckman (1965), once the group is formed it follows a set of successive stages and these are forming, storming, norming, performing and adjourning.

Forming

Forming is described as a testing period, where group members get to know each other and start to establish certain basic ground rules. These would include discussing behaviour which is permissible and what is not permissible to exhibit. This stage suggests that members adopt a certain behaviour that would be described as rather superficial in that the members are not fully trusting of each other.

Storming

Storming has an element of competing for the attractive roles and this can lead to intragroup conflicts. There may be pairing and subgroup formation. Members may discover their individual needs to be different to one another. There may also be competition for the leadership role.

Norming

Norming sees a common perspective emerging and the foundation is set for the group to perform. Arguments are settled and decisions are made based on shared rules. Members develop emotional attachment to each other. Group cohesion is established and members feel able to express their feelings and opinions.

Performing

Performing emphasises getting on with the task at hand and the group focuses on working towards the goals.

Adjourning

Adjourning is the stage where the group comes to its end. The task is finished, all the goals have been achieved or not as the case may be, and so the group disbands. Depending on the time the group has been together, members may choose to stay together for social reasons.

From Yalom's (1985) perspective groups travel through the stages of

- orientation
- conflict and
- cohesiveness

Orientation is the initial stage and members have two set tasks to engage in.

Orientation

1   They need to establish a way to accomplish the task.
2   They work towards comfort, meaning and pleasure of being in the group.

There is still an element of hesitancy in group members' behaviour and getting to know one another is one of its main features. Other activities include searching for things they have in common with other members of the group.

Conflict is the second stage of group formation and this is centred around preoccupation with dominance, control and power. Conflict emerges between members or members and leader. This is similar to Tuckman and Jensen's storming stage.

Conflict

Cohesiveness is the third stage of group formation and shows an element of greater trust, high morale and more disclosure. Members become more committed to one another.

Cohesiveness

Bion's perspective on groups

Bion's (1961) perspective on groups suggests that the emotional states of the group somehow dictates its dynamics. There are three types of emotional states and these are

- aggressiveness, hostility, and fear
- optimism and hopeful anticipation
- helplessness or awe

Bion's argument is that when members are in each of these emotional states, they behave as if they share some beliefs which generate these emotions. If for example the group is in an aggressive, hostile or fearful state, then its members will behave as if to avoid something by fighting or running away from it. Similarly when the group is in an optimistic and hopeful mood, its members will behave as if to preserve the group by finding strength. When the group is in a helpless state, its members search for support from outside. Each of these three emotional states are referred to as Basic Assumption Cultures. This suggests that there are three basic assumption groups, these being

Basic assumption cultures

Aggressiveness, hostility and fear = basic assumption fight–flight
Optimism and hopeful anticipation = basic assumption pairing
Helplessness or awe = basic assumption dependency

Bion's view indicates a central role for the leader and each basic assumption group will search for a specific type of leader to fulfil its needs, for example a fight–flight group will look for someone who will help them to pursue this goal. The role of the leader in these situations is extremely important.

Factors influencing group behaviour

According to McGregor (1960) the effectiveness of any group depends on the following factors:

- Atmosphere. The recipe for effectiveness is based on a relaxed and comfortable atmosphere, free from tension, where everyone is interested and involved.
- Discussion. This is focused and everyone participates.
- Objectives. These are clearly understood and accepted by group members.
- Listening. Members will actively listen to one another. Everyone has an opportunity to express, members do not seem to be afraid to say what they feel.
- Disagreement. If there are any disagreements, the group is comfortable to deal with it, there is no indication of avoidance behaviour.
- Decisions. These are made by consensus but majority rules however do not always apply, the group will explore other avenues and issues which will best serve their purpose.
- Criticism. This is kept open, there is no hidden agenda and members are comfortable.
- Feelings. These are expressed freely.
- Action. This is clearly defined and members are fully committed.
- Leadership. This is flexible, and there is no domination by the leader. There is no struggle for power.
- Self-conscious. The group is aware of its modes of operation and it frequently reflects on what has happened.

Role functions

Role can be defined as a 'set of behaviours that is expected or and/or displayed by the individual who occupies a particular position in a group's structure' (Barker *et al.*, 1979, p.162).

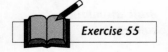 *Exercise 55*

Reflect on the various groups of which you are a member and identify the different roles you have or had.

Reflecting on some of the groups I belong to, I can conclude the following roles: Husband, Father, Son, Lecturer, Psychologist, Nurse, Examiner, Supervisor and so on. Within each of those groups my roles are well defined and are qualitatively different from one another. Your roles could be similarly defined. Having said that who actually defines the roles one plays in one's different group? According to Thibault and Kelly (1959), there are four different criteria for roles and these are:

1   Prescribed roles. This is a way in which one is expected to conform according to societal norms.
2   Subjective roles. This is basically what the individual perceives to be his or her roles.
3   Enacted roles. This is the role which the individual actually plays. The focus is on the displayed behaviour.
4   Functionally requisite role. The emphasis is on the functional value of either the prescribed or the enacted roles.

If any group is to survive, roles must be fulfilled. Penland and Fine (1974, p.71) state 'as a group need arises, someone in the group invariably assumes a role that will fulfil that need'. Having said that it is also possible that one of the group's members may take on a blocking role, which would then hinder the group growth and development. This is called sabotage and to keep the flavour of self-awareness, perhaps you could have a go at Exercise 56.

Think of the numerous ways you can actually sabotage your group. I will start you off with, 'I can sabotage my/this group by whispering to a colleague next to me during a group discussion'. This exercise is much more revealing in a classroom situation, where each member would make his or her statement to the rest of the group.

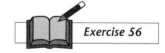

Exercise 56

Penland and Fine's analysis of roles show three broad categories.

a   Group task roles
b   Group building and maintaining roles
c   Individual roles

Group task roles are based on the task which the group has to undertake. The emphasis is on facilitating and co-ordinating group effort in identifying and dealing with problems. Any of the following roles may be played by various members of the group.

Group task roles

•   Initiator–contributor. Member offers new ideas or a different way of looking at the group's problem
•   Information seeker. Member asks for information in search for clarification regarding the group's problem
•   Opinion seeker. Member asks for clarification regarding the value of what's proposed
•   Information giver. Member offers information which is relevant to the group's problem

- Opinion giver. Member gives his or her opinion of what he or she thinks should be the group's value
- Elaborator. Member explains a rationale for his or her suggestion
- Co-ordinator. Member tries bringing other members' ideas together
- Orienter. Member defines the position of the group according to its goals
- Evaluator. Member offers a judgement of the group's achievement in comparison to its goals
- Energiser. Member steers the group into action
- Procedural technician. Member does certain things for the group
- Recorder. Member records minutes of the meetings and the decisions which the group makes

Group building and maintaining roles

Group building and maintaining roles which are centred on the functioning of the group as a group. Changes are made to the group's way of working if necessary, the intention is to strengthen and regulate the group. The following roles are included.

- Encourager. Member accepts and praises the others for contributing
- Harmoniser. Member smoothes things out in times of conflict
- Compromiser. Member admits to his or her mistake and alters his or her position to suit
- Gate-keeper and expediter. Member ensures everyone has a chance to voice his or her opinion
- Group observer and commentator. Member keeps a record on group process
- Follower. Member remains a passive follower throughout.

Individual roles

There is an element of focusing on members' individual needs, group needs take second place. This could lead to conflict between members. The roles include

- Aggressor, who functions purely by being destructive in numerous ways
- Blocker, who adopts an attitude of negativism. This is similar to a saboteur
- Recognition-seeker, who sets out to attract attention to him/herself through numerous strategies
- Self-confessor, who uses the group to off-load personal issues
- Playboy, who never gets involved and remains in isolation
- Dominator, who seeks to control through manipulative means
- Help-seeker, who asks for sympathy
- Special-interest-pleader, who speaks for the others, like the minority group

Penland and Fine note that these roles are not confined to one particular member and as such they are not static nor consistent. This would suggest that permanently labelling members would not be valuable, but it may be sufficient to just recognise the role being played at a particular time by a particular member.

Leadership and leadership style

It could be argued that if a group is to be effective, its leader must be accepted by its members. Shaw (1981) states that the leadership role is one of the most important roles associated with positions in group structure. So what then is leadership? Embroiled within the concept of leadership is the leader. According to Bass (1981), leadership can have numerous facets and these can range from being the focus of group processes to an instrument of goal achievement.

Leadership as a focus of group processes places the leader in the central position where communication is controlled. Bass (1981) reflected Krech and Crutchfield's (1948) sentiment and suggests that the position which the leader occupies makes him or her a primary agent for determining group structure, group atmosphere, group goals, group ideology, and group activities.

Leadership as a focus of group processes

Leadership as personality and its effects implies a set of significant traits which the leader needs to have in order to be effective in that central position. Some of these traits include charisma, social boldness, highly dominant in times of crisis, and empathic understanding.

Leadership as personality and its effects

According to Munson (1921), leadership is the art of inducing compliance in that the position suggests an element of being able to deal with group members in such a way so as to achieve the most with the least friction and greatest co-operation.

Leadership as the art of inducing compliance

Leadership as a power relation implies that the leader is the one with the power to influence group members into action. Bass (1981, p.12) states, 'it can be observed that some leaders more than others tend to transform any opportunity into an overt power relationship'.

Leadership as a power relation

Leadership as an instrument of goal achievement is often used to define the term leadership. For example Hollander (1978) sees leadership as the process through which one member of a specific group, that is its leader, influences other group members towards the attainment of specific group goals. Tannenbaum and Massarik (1957) define leadership as an interpersonal influence, which is exercised in situations and directed, through the communication process, toward the attainment of specified goal or goals.

Leadership as an instrument of goal achievement

Whichever way one defines leadership, one factor remains obvious and that is the issue of 'influence'. Influence is geared towards the achievement of a certain goal. A leader therefore is the person with such an influence. Shaw (1981, p.319) defines a leader as a 'member of the group who exerts positive influence over other group members, or as the member who exerts more positive influence over others than they exert over him or her'. The word positive is taken to mean the direction which is preferred by the leader.

Leadership as the exercise of influence

A leader can emerge as a result of his or her forceful personality, or a leader can be appointed by the group members. Obviously the latter choice would present better group dynamics. Having said that it does not necessarily follow that every group will have a leader, it is possible to have a leaderless group. In this situation all or most of the group members would contribute towards achieving its goals. Barker *et al.* (1979, p.227) offer a further scenario where 'leadershipless' exists and this would mean 'an absence of action which is moving the group towards its goal.' Here obviously the group may not be as successful as other groups that have a leader. Numerous factors contribute to who becomes a leader. These include the following:

- personal characteristics
- individual behaviour
- skills, knowledge, and attitudes
- characteristics of the task
- environment
- group needs

Natural born leader

Are leaders born or does one acquire the skills of leadership? This is an interesting question indeed. Penington (1986, p.233) states 'historically and traditionally a leader has been viewed as a person possessing a distinct set of personality characteristics'. On the face of it, there is a general impression that there are certain traits which make a great leader. Baron and Byrne (1991) point to such great leaders as Alexander the Great, Queen Elizabeth I, Abraham Lincoln, and suggest that they were different in many aspects to ordinary people. There does not seem to be any strong evidence to support the belief that leaders are born. Early research however er concluded from the 'great person or trait theory' that great leaders do possess certain key traits that distinguish them from other people. This is purely conjecture because there is no research evidence to support this belief.

Leadership styles

Shaw (1981) states that even casual observation of leaders at work shows that there are differences in the styles of leadership, for example some would give orders, make all decisions without consulting the group or even regardless of what the rest of the members think, and demand obedience. Whilst others are considerate, ask for members' co-operation, consult members for their opinions before making decisions. The style of leadership therefore is significant to the dynamics of the group.

Lewin *et al.* (1939) identified three styles of leadership and these are:

- authoritarian
- democratic
- laissez-faire

Authoritarian style   The authoritarian style of leadership would be exemplified by the scenario of basically going it alone and doing everything without consulting the rest of the group. The authoritarian leader would demand obedience and everything would be structured according to how he or she sees the situation. According to Bass (1981), the authoritarian leader dictates what is to be done and is unconcerned about group members' need for autonomy and development. Authoritarian leaders are task orientated and as such are concerned with getting the 'job done'. The leader is personal in praise and aloof from the group members.

Although authoritarian leadership style comes across as negative, it has to be said that there are advantages and disadvantages to its group dynamics and the achievement of group goal. With this in mind list some advantages and disadvantages of this style of leadership as applicable to your workplace.

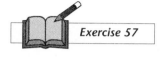

Exercise 57

A democratic style of leadership is more flexible and 'shared the decision making with subordinates and was concerned about their needs to contribute to deciding on what was to be done' (Bass, 1981, p.293). Democratic leaders emphasised social closeness and interpersonal relations.

Democratic style

List some of the advantages and disadvantages of this style of leadership style in relation to your workplace.

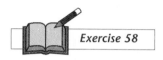

Exercise 58

Laissez-faire style of leadership is characterised by the leader allowing members to do as they wish. He or she would take on a more passive role. The group does not receive any feedback from the laissez-faire leader regarding the task. Laissez-faire leaders do not attempt to influence their subordinates and basically have no confidence in their own ability. 'They bury themselves in paper work and . . . . stay away from subordinates, set no clear goals toward which they may work, and do not make decisions to help their group to make decisions. They tend to let things drift' (Bass, 1981, p.394).

Laissez-faire style

Consider what you feel are some of the advantages and disadvantages of the laissez-faire styles of leadership in relation to your workplace.

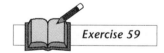

Exercise 59

Look closely at all three styles of leadership and consider which health care scenarios you feel warrant specific styles of leadership. For example an authoritarian style leadership may be more appropriate in an emergency situation, where one person needs to take control and dictate to others what to do. Think along these lines.

In a study conducted by Lewin *et al.* (1939), four comparable groups of 10-year-old boys were observed as they performed a task (carving models from bars of soap) under the three different styles of leadership. The experiment was structured in such a way as to ensure that each group experienced a 3-week period under the leadership style of an authoritarian, democratic and laissez-faire adult. Four adult leaders were involved and each adult was prepared for all the three leadership styles. This meant that each group had a different leader after each period of 3 weeks. The displayed characteristics of each of the leaders were as follows.

- The authoritarian leader would determine everything that needs to be done. Every instruction and ways of behaving were dictated. Praise and criticism were subjective.
- The democratic leader would allow the group to make decisions and members were free to work with anyone they wanted to. Praise and criticism was based objectively.
- The laissez-faire leader would not participate in the activity and the group was free to do what they wanted. Information was given as and when asked for and feedback was infrequent.

The results showed that there were significant differences in behaviour in response to the different styles of leadership for example.

- Hostility and aggression were higher under authoritarian as compared to democratic leaders.
- Scapegoating occurred more frequently in authoritarian than in either of the other styles.
- The product was qualitatively superior in the democratic groups than in the other two groups.
- Morale was by far higher in the democratic groups.

From this study, although fairly dated, one can conclude that leadership style is significant to the group process and dynamics. The implication is that a democratic style of leadership outweighs the other two styles in terms of rapport and relationship. Having said that perhaps the most important element in the concept of leadership style is the situation one finds oneself in. In many ways it is the situation that ought to decide which style of leadership one needs to adopt. With this in mind perhaps an eclectic style is one that any leader should go for.

Reflect on your own style of leadership and establish the kind of leader you are.

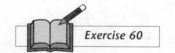

Exercise 60

Check out also the appropriateness of your style in context of the situation you are in.

Your findings may enhance your awareness of the way you lead or care for your patients.

Communication and leadership

Bavelas (1950) used five networks of communication from an experiment which he conducted with five subjects. Each subject was given a set of cards (poker hands) and the object of the game was to find the best poker hand from the combined cards of all the five members. The subjects communicated only by written messages. The five channels of communication were circle, wheel, all-channel, chain and 'Y' or yoke.

Circle communication network

The circle network of communication suggests that each member has an equal opportunity to send messages to and receive messages from the member to both his or her right and left side (see Figure 14.1).

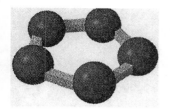

Figure 14.1
The circle pattern of communication where each member has the opportunity of interacting with at least two members of the group

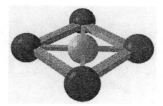

Figure 14.2
The wheel communication network suggests equal access to the leader who is in the centre

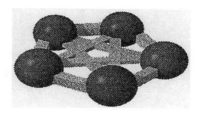

Figure 14.3
The open channel of communication suggests every member has an equal chance of communicating with each other and is indicative of a democratic style of communication

The wheel network of communication shows four members with equal chances of communicating with the member in the centre (see Figure 14.2).

The all-channel communication network is an open channel communication, where each member has an equal chance of communicating with any other member in the group. This particular method of communication would seem to be most desired in a cohesive group (see Figure 14.3).

The chain communication network means that any member could in fact send messages to the member in the centre but all messages will have to be relayed by the two members who are nearest to the member in the centre (see Figure 14.4).

The 'Y' communication network is such that only three members would in fact have direct communication with the member in the centre, the rest would have to communicate to the member in the centre through one of the other members (see Figure 14.5).

Wheel communication network

All-channel communication network

Chain communication network

'Y' or yoke communication network

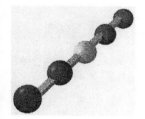

Figure 14.4
The chain channel of communication suggests a linear system of communication and members have to interact via other members in order to communicate with every one

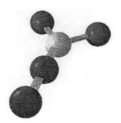

Figure 14.5
The 'Y' channel of communication shows similar dynamics to that of the chain channel in that one of its members has to communicate via another member in order to reach the member in the middle

Of the five channels of communication, the all-channel network offers the best opportunity for every member to have their say and this could be one of the most important factors in group cohesion and fulfilment of a group's goal. This would suggest that one of the prerequisites for effective leadership is the skill of being able to freely communicate with every member of the group. Effective communication holds the key to a stable group life, successful group dynamics and hence reduced conflicts. Interpersonal conflict is the topic of discussion in Chapter 15.

References

Barker, L., Cegala, D.L., Kibler, R.J. and Wahlers, K.J. (1979). *An Introduction to Small Group Communication*. Englewood Cliff, NJ: Prentice-Hall.

Baron, R.A. and Byrne, D. (1991). *Social Psychology. Understanding Human Interaction*. Boston, London, Toronto, Sydney, Tokyo, Singapore: Allyn and Bacon.

Bass, B.M. (1981). *Stogdill's Handbook of Leadership. A Survey of Theory and Research*, revised and expanded edn. New York: The Free Press. London: Collier MacMillan.

Bavelas, A. (1950). 'Communication patterns in task-oriented groups.' *Journal of the Acoustical Society of America* **22**, 725–730.

Bion, W.R. (1961). *Experiences in Groups*. New York: Basic Books.

Blumberg, H., Hare, P., Kent, V. and Davies, M. (1983). *Small Groups and Social Interaction*, Vol. 2. Chichester: John Wiley and Sons.

Hollander, E.P. (1978). *Leadership Dynamics: A Practical Guide to Effective Relationships*. New York: Free Press.

Krech, D. and Crutchfield, R.S. (1948). *Theory and Problems of Social Psychology*. New York: McGraw-Hill.

Lewin, K., Lippitt, R. and White, R. (1939). 'Patterns of aggressive behaviour in experimentally created "social Climates."' *Journal of Social Psychology*, **10**, 271–299.

McGregor, D.M. (1960). *The Human Side of Enterprise*. New York: McGraw-Hill.

Munson, E.L. (1921). *The Management of Men*. New York: Holt, Rinehart and Winston.

Penington, D.C. (1986). *Essential Social Psychology*. London, Edward Arnold.

Penland, P.R. and Fine, S.F. (1974). *Group Dynamics and Individual Development*. New York: Marcel Dekker, Inc.

Schutz, W. (1958). *FIRO: A Three Dimensional Theory of Interpersonal Behaviour*. New York: Holt, Rinehart and Winston.

Schutz, W. (1983). 'A theory of small groups.' In: Blumberg, H., Hare, P., Kent, V. and Davies, M. (Eds) *Small Groups and Social Interaction*, Vol. 2. Chichester: John Wiley and Sons.

Shaw, M.E. (1981). *Group Dynamics. The Psychology of Small Group Behaviour*. New York: McGraw-Hill.

Tannenbaum, R. and Massarik, F. (1957). *Leadership and Organisation: A Behavioural Science Approach*. New York: McGraw-Hill.

Thibaut, J.W. and Kelly, H.H. (1959). *The Social Psychology of Groups*. New York, London, Sydney: John Wiley and Sons.

Tuckman, B.W. (1965). 'Developmental sequence in small groups.' *Psychological Bulletin*, **63**, 384–399.

Yalom, I.D. (1985). T*he Theory and Practice of Group Psychotherapy*. New York: Basic Books.

Interpersonal conflict: dynamics, resolutions and self-awareness

15

Objectives

After reading this chapter you should be able to:

1   Explain what a conflict is
2   List some of the characteristics of a conflict
3   List and explain some of the levels at which conflict can take place
4   Describe the conflict process
5   Recognise some of the ways of dealing with a conflict
6   Describe some of the basic rules of behaviour for the professional carer
7   List some of the basic rules of behaviour for the recipient of care
8   Explain some of the implications of conflict at work

Conflict and behaviour

The need to learn the art of communication could not be any greater than in helping to resolve conflict between two or more people. To be in conflict suggests being at odds with one another. A person's thoughts, feelings and actions are in direct contradiction with others. According to Filley (1975), a conflict would arise if the interests of the parties concerned are mutually exclusive. This suggests that one person benefits to the detriment of the other person, an example would be political parties, each with their own ideology and obviously in direct contradiction with the other parties. There are at least two different kinds of conflict, these are competitive and disruptive.

Competitive conflict can easily be observed in political parties, where victory for one means defeat for the others. The parties strive for goals which are wholly incompatible with one another.

Competitive conflict

Disruptive conflict is not about winning, the emphasis instead is on defeating, harming or driving away the opponent.

Disruptive conflict

Very often there is an interplay between competitive and destructive conflict. Filley (1975, p.3) states that from experience one can conclude that conflicts are usually distributed along a continuum between those that are competitive and those that are disruptive. Losing could trigger anger feelings, and these could escalate to aggressive and violent behaviour.

Characteristics of conflict

The characteristics of a conflict are summarised as follows.

- There are at least two parties involved in some sort of interaction
- The values and/or goals are mutually exclusive to one another
- The focus of the interaction is aimed to defeat, harm or suppress the opponent or to be the victor
- Both parties' actions are in direct opposition to one another
- Each party seeks to create an imbalance of power in their own favour

Levels of conflict

According to Rapoport (1960), there are basically three levels at which a conflict can take place. These are:

a   Fights, where force is involved and the prime objective is to incapacitate or eliminate the opponent
b   Games, where the purpose is to win without eliminating the opponent
c   Debates, where the objective is to change the opinion of your opponent

The dynamics of conflict

Conflict is not a static process. Conflict would always involve two or more people with a set of attitude, values, beliefs, goals and with any other attributes which are to some extent, opposite to each other (see Figure 15.1). Suppose carer Jim believes that patients should have free and easy access to their personal records. Carer John on the other hand believes the opposite, that is, all records should be strictly confidential. The situation which develops would suggest that both Jim and John are heading in completely different directions. If John decide to co-operate with Jim, then a conflict will be avoided. A conflict situation would emerge if both stick to their beliefs. According to Sisson and Ackeroff (1966) a conflict is negative co-operation. Here therefore the outcome of Jim's attitude, beliefs, values and goals will be influenced by John's attitude, beliefs, values and goals. Similarly, John's outcome will be influenced by Jim. Sisson and Ackeroff

Figure 15.1

A conflict situation as a result of two opposing sets of ideas working against each other

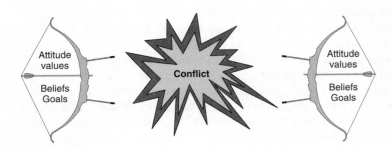

further believe that conflict and co-operation are not necessarily symmetrical. What they mean is that, if I am in conflict with you, it does not necessarily follow that you are in conflict with me. It may well be that you are co-operating with me.

The conflict process

Filley says that there are six steps to the process of conflict, these are:

1 the antecedents
2 cognitive appraisal
3 affective appraisal
4 behavioural manifestation
5 conflict resolution or suppression
6 resolution aftermath

Antecedents basically mean the events leading to the conflict. Some of the factors which contribute to conflicts include:

Antecedents

* Lack of clear boundaries, for example two people in the same department may have similar job descriptions and as a result confusion may rise as to who is doing what.
* Conflict of interest, for example I am travelling in the car with one of my sons and I want to listen to my favourite Celine Dion cassette and my son wishes to play his Bon Jovi, Alanis Morrisette or Sheryl Crow. We both have our own interests. Here however I can easily resolve this conflict by reminding my son that, in my car we do it my way. A true conflict of interest however may not be that simple to resolve.
* Lack of understanding between two people, for example you have arranged to meet your partner at 2.15 p.m. Unfortunately on arriving at the proposed destination, you discover that your partner had in fact been waiting for half an hour, under the impression that you had said 1.45 p.m.
* Dependence and reliance on one party in a relationship.
* Increase in hierarchical structure and numerous tiers in organisations.
* Too many members involved in decision making. This is a case of too many cooks spoil the broth.
* Consensus is essential for moving forward. If we have a group of 10 people, it would be very difficult to have everybody agreeing with one another.
* Strict rules and regulations are imposed on members.
* Unresolved prior conflicts.

The argument in cognitive appraisal is that if a situation is inaccurately perceived, the likelihood is that conflict will result. Similarly if no solution or compromise is perceived, conflict will escalate. If a situation is per-

Cognitive appraisal

ceived as a 'potential conflict', then the parties concerned could take steps to avoid it. If on the other hand both parties are unaware of a conflict situation, then conflict may not develop. Filley (1975, p.12) states, 'failure to identify potentially conflictive conditions may prevent conflicts from developing'. This has the sentiment of 'ignorance is bliss'.

Affective experience

The affective experience focuses on the feeling aspects of both parties. If the nature of the interaction is personalised, by 'blaming the other' for the feelings experienced by one another, then conflict will result. If the interaction is depersonalised, that is, blaming the exhibited behaviour, conflict may not occur. This gives the message, 'as a person, you are ok, but your behaviour is upsetting'.

Behavioural manifestation

In behavioural manifestation, the question is one of intent, for example, do you intend to prevent me from achieving my goals? If I perceive this as a 'yes', then conflict will escalate. If you accidentally block me, then there is a slight chance that conflict may develop.

Conflict resolution or suppression

Conflict resolution or suppression is the stage where the conflict is either resolved or placed on hold. The resolution of conflict is dependent on what happened in behavioural manifestation. Resolution will only take place if both parties are prepared to collaborate. There are many unresolved conflicts and these in themselves may not be problematic, but forced attempts at resolving them may fuel the conflicts. An attitude of 'let sleeping dogs lie' is probably the only solution.

Resolution aftermath

Resolution aftermath will depend on how the conflict was resolved. Was there a winner and a loser? If there was a winner, the other party would be left with a feeling of defeat and loss. This in itself can be an antecedent for future conflict. From the positive side, both parties may have resolved the conflict amicably and with good feelings.

Prisoner's dilemma

Imagine the following scenario which is based on Rapoport's (1974) account of the prisoner's dilemma. You and your friend have been convicted of the same crime and are taken into custody and placed in separate cells. The police do not have enough evidence to convict you or your friend for the crime, they do however have sufficient evidence to convict both of you for a minor crime and this carries the sentence of 1 year imprisonment. The police decide to offer each of you the following deal.

1   Confess and you go free but your friend would then get the maximum sentence which is 10 years in prison.
2   Maintain your silence and accept the consequence of 1 year in prison, provided of course your friend does not confess.

This leaves you with the following scenarios:

a   You confess, you walk free but your friend gets 10 years
b   You maintain your silence but your friend confesses, he walks free and you get 10 years
c   You confess but your friend also confesses, so you both get 10 years
d   You and your friend maintain your silence, so you both get 1 year each

You now find yourself in a state of conflict. How do you deal with such a conflict?

Dealing with conflict

Basically any conflict can be dealt with, in any one of the three possible ways and these are win–lose, lose–lose and win–win.

In a win–lose scenario, there is one winner and one loser, and this is **Win–lose** based on the issue of power. This is obvious in any type of conflict between an employer and his or her employee, where the boss always wins. In the prisoner's dilemma if one confesses, the other does not, the confessor is the winner.

According to Edelmann (1993), some of the factors which are likely to contribute a win–lose scenario are:

a   Believing that one person must lose for the other one to win
b   Lack of honesty and openness
c   Lack of self-awareness regarding one's negative point
d   Lack of recognition of the other person's positive points
e   Tit for tat game, in the vein of 'an eye for an eye'
f   Failure to listen
g   Blaming the other person
h   An eagerness to criticise

In a lose–lose scenario, there is no winner and neither parties are pre- **Lose–lose** pared to compromise their position and perhaps avoid any personal con- frontation regarding the particular issue. The lose–lose scenario in the pris- oner's dilemma is when both confess.

A win–win scenario is based on a problem solving approach where both **Win–win** parties are satisfied. In the prisoner's dilemma even without the ability to communicate with each other, both could win and all they have to do is to maintain their silence. They would still have to go to prison but it would have been worst for at least one of them.

Think of some examples for each of the win–lose, lose–lose and win–win scenarios.

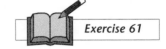
Exercise 61

In the win–lose strategy, you could think of examples regarding the fol- lowing:

• Power issue in terms of either intellectual or physical
• Failure to respond, for example no one responds to my suggestion for starting off each session with a warm up exercise
• Majority wins, some poor souls will be left disappointed
• Minority wins, like if you happen to be the boss or your face fits. Or in a group of 10 people three or four people are loud and forceful, the rest may feel threatened and decide not to get involved

In the lose-lose strategy, you could think of examples such as:

- Compromising your values
- One party accepts some sort of bribe to lose
- Fight till you drop

Factors which contribute to the win–lose scenario are similar to the lose–lose strategy. For the win–win scenario, the focus is on where both parties benefit from the approach they have adopted to resolve the conflict. Edelmann (1993) suggests four steps which contribute to a positive outcome for both parties and these are:

- Recognising that a problem exists
- Understanding of each other's perspective
- Discussing the problem and its possible solution
- Resolving the problem so that both benefit

Rules of behaviour for professional carer/helper

Edelmann (1993) has listed a set of rules of professional relationships, which he argues contributes to the avoidance of conflict. Some of these rules are related to behaviour of:

1   Professional caregivers
2   Patients/clients

An attempt is made here at summarising Edelmann's sentiments. The professional carer or helper should:

- Listen to the patients
- Inform and check for understanding
- Offer appropriate support and counselling
- Refer to others if needs arise
- Be genuine and show respect
- Maintain confidentiality
- Avoid publicly criticising the patient
- Avoid overinvolvement to the point of sexual intimacy
- Not engage in inappropriate self-disclosure

Rules of behaviour for patients

The patient should

- Ask for clarification
- Follow advice and instruction
- Provide any information which contributes to his or her well-being

- Be genuine
- Not be overdemanding
- Respect the carer's privacy

Conflict at work

Edelmann (1993) reckons that people on average spend about 100 000 hours at work during their lives. This suggests that one spends a great deal of the time working with or in the company of others. When conflict does arise in the workplace, the lives of those involved can be extremely difficult. Although the conflicts may occur at work, the individuals tend to take the problem home with them, thus disrupting both their lives and the lives of those people around them like their mothers, fathers, husbands, wives, children, boyfriends and girlfriends. Sometimes a lot of displacements go on. Edelmann (1993) identifies the following factors which contribute to making lives stressful.

1 The nature of the job itself, for example we may be asked to do too much and what is worse is watching your colleagues doing much less than you.
2 The level of responsibility you may be asked to take on is far more than you are able to deal with. Worse still, you may be asked to do something that you do not enjoy.
3 Lack of consultation, the classic one is, being volunteered in one's absence.
4 Lack of opportunity to grow and develop, as in thwarted ambition.
5 Relationship (intimate) with one's boss, colleagues, clients, patients and students

Look at your own workplace and identify the factors which may give rise to conflicts. Identify the effects these may have on you.

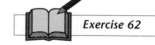 Exercise 62

Although hard to believe you may be surprised to read that there is such a thing as positive effects of conflict. These include:

- Strengthening a relationship
- Development of greater trust
- Increased productivity
- Job satisfaction

The negative effects of conflict include:

- Low morale
- Little or no job satisfaction
- Alienation
- Physical illnesses
- Mental health problems

Conflict and self-awareness

In any interaction, as Berne (1964) illustrated, a complementary exchange of ideas is productive, whereas, a crossed or ulterior transaction leads to a block in communication. Any attempt at resolving a conflict therefore has to have a complementary transaction as its basis. By its very nature, conflict suggests, 'being at odds with one another', as for example if both you and I are driving towards each other on a very narrow country lane, where there is only room for one car to go through. Neither of us wants to reverse into a lay-by to allow the other to pass. A conflict situation therefore develops. Although in this situation the possible outcomes could be: winner and loser, loser and loser, and winner and winner, provided in this instance both parties are prepared to communicate.

The whole concept of conflict offers an insight into the fact that if two people are in conflict with one another, each will want to win at the expense of the other. One way of resolving the conflict would be for both individuals to engage in empathic listening, allowing each the opportunity to express his or her thoughts and feelings. Although it is recommended that one tries to resolve a conflict, it needs to be acknowledged that sometimes this may not be possible. In such an instance, agree to disagree might be the best policy to adopt. From a health care perspective, lack of self-awareness and lack of communication are two of the most frequent causes of conflict. Self-awareness can prevent or resolve conflict, by generating empathic understanding on the part of carers. Carers can examine their own set of attitudes, values and beliefs with a view to respecting the attitudes, values and beliefs of the patients. Interpersonal communication remains a focal point of conflict resolution. Effective interpersonal skills however are prerequisites to the concept of caring. Section III deals with some of the issues of interpersonal communication and health care practice.

References

Berne, E. (1964). *Games People Play; The Psychology of Human Relationships.* London: Penguin Books.

Edelmann, R.J. (1993). *Interpersonal Conflicts at Work.* Leicester: British Psychological Society.

Filley, A.C. (1975). *Interpersonal Conflict Resolution.* Oxford: Scott, Foresman and Company.

Rapoport, A. (1960). *Fights, Games, and Debates.* Ann Arbor: University of Michigan Press.

Rapoport, A. (Ed.) (1974). *Game Theory as a Theory of Conflict Resolution.* Boston: D. Reidl Publishing Company.

Sisson, R.L. and Ackeroff, R.L. (1966). 'Toward a theory of the dynamics of conflict.' In: Mudd, S. (Ed.) *Conflict Resolution and World Education.* The Hague: D.R.W. Junk.

Interpersonal skills and practice

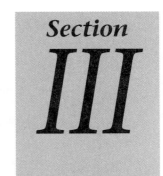

Introduction

Communication is probably one of the most researched subjects in the field of human behaviour. Having said that, it is still not any easier to articulate its meaning. It is not as simple as 'you talk to me and I talk to you'. It could be argued that interpersonal communication holds the key to whether sexual intercourse is a pleasurable experience or rape. A rather crude and insensitive way of introducing this section, one may say, however from a purely practical point of view, sexual intercourse is a pleasurable experience when both parties concerned have a common understanding as to what they both want. If one party wants to hold hands, the other party wants to kiss, communication is not about holding hands and kissing. It is much more than that, it is about finding a common understanding between two people. This common understanding is crucial to whether an individual is successful at communicating or not. We may delude ourselves into believing that we all have the gift of communicating, sadly though, we are not born with the ability to understand each other, it is a skill that we have to learn. The ability to understand one another is amongst the numerous skills one needs in order to establish effective interpersonal communication. Interpersonal communication is inextricably linked with interpersonal skills. There is a positive correlation between interpersonal skills and communication, good interpersonal skills lead to effective communication and inadequate or inappropriate interpersonal skills mean ineffective communication.

Interpersonal skills

What are interpersonal skills? Interpersonal skills are those skills which one needs in order to communicate effectively with another person or a group of people. The key element of interpersonal skills is self-awareness, and this filters through every single micro-component of person to person relationships. These components include warmth, acceptance, genuineness, empathy, listening, attending and responding. Listening, attending and responding fall in the realm of verbal, non-verbal, and paralanguage (see Figure 16.1).

Figure 16.1
*Micro-components of
communication with self-
awareness as its focal point*

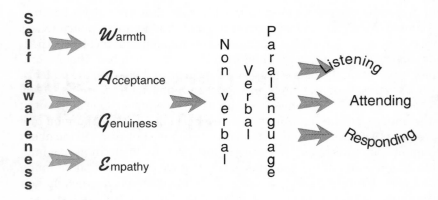

According to Johnson and Johnson (1991, p.106) communication is
much more than just the exchange of words. It is a process whereby
'everyone receives, sends, interprets, and infers all at the same time. There
is no beginning and no end; all communication involves persons sending
one another symbols to which certain meanings are attached.' People
interact with one another both verbally and non-verbally, communication
therefore is only possible if both parties adopt the same ways of relating to
these verbal or non-verbal experiences.

Laswell's (1960) model of communication simplifies the concept to
reflect the sentiment of 'who says what to whom through what channel
with what effect'.

- Who (sender)
- Says what (message)
- How (channel/method)
- To whom (receiver)
- With what effect (response)

**When it goes wrong,
blame the sender**

In this respect, if I was to send a verbal message to you and it does not
have the desired effect on you, I could not say that we have communicated. According to Johnson and Johnson, for interpersonal communication
to take place, a message, sent by a person to another person, must consciously affect the receiver's behaviour. The effectiveness of the communication therefore depends on whether the sender's intended message is
interpreted in the same way as intended by the receiver. Ley (1988) says
that if a message is not understood by its intended audience, it would
make more sense to blame the sender. This may seem harsh, but which
shall we go for, 'blame the patient for not understanding or remembering
the information' or 'blame the carer for not making the information clear
enough for the patient to understand'. I would look ridiculous if I were to
tell you that it was my car's fault for running out of petrol. Scapegoating
the patient for one's inability to communicate properly is not something
to boast about. It could be said that the patient has good reasons to forget
or misinterpret the information they are given. For example they could be
so preoccupied with their own problems that they are unable to take it all

in and some carers could use so much jargon that the patient becomes confused. As Ley said, some patients thought that a lumbar puncture was an operation to drain the lungs, and others thought that incubation period was the length of stay the child would have to stay in bed. These examples suggest that the blame rests with the carers and not with the patients.

An overview of the mechanics of communication goes some way towards explaining how messages can be misinterpreted. One of the most used models of communication was developed in 1947, by Shannon and Weaver (1949), who according to Berlo (1960) were not even talking about human communication, they were in fact referring to electronic communication. Social and behavioural scientists have capitalised on Shannon and Weaver's model, showing how and what really happens when human communication is in progress. According to Shannon and Weaver, there are five ingredients in communication and these are:

- a source (where the message comes from)
- a transmitter (who is sending out the source's message)
- a signal (how is the message sent)
- a receiver (who accepts the message) and
- a destination (where is the message going).

Most of the social and behavioural theorists agree on one basic model of communication. This model reflects some of the sentiments which have already been explored, there are still some other ingredients which need to be considered. In its entirety, the most popular communication model which is used is as follows.

1   Sender (self)
2   Encoder (converting thought into message)
3   Channel (verbal, non-verbal, both verbal and non-verbal)
4   Decoder (interpretation of message)
5   Receiver (other/others)

Transposing this communication model into an interpersonal situation will possibly result in the following scenario.

Let us assume that the starting point of any communication is with self. I have a thought in my head, I convert this thought into a coded message in the form of any of my senses (either verbal, non-verbal). Before you receive this message, you have to recognise the coded signal (through some of your senses), then interpret the signal and when you have the intended meaning of my thought, only then, will we have communicated. This is an enormous task, a task which is further complicated by an individual's intrapersonal dynamics. Other influential factors which may affect the process of communication include, one's interpersonal skills and abilities to interact with others, one's knowledge, one's social system and one's culture. This section will deal with some of these issues, such as trust, disclosure, feedback, assertiveness, in relation to health care delivery. The concept of helping is explored through Egan's (1990), Brammer's (1988) models, and Heron's (1990) concept of Six Category Intervention Analysis.

The focus will be on some of the micro-skills of therapeutic communication. A reminder here that therapeutic communication is taken to mean any interaction which leads to the enhancement of the client's growth, development and autonomy, so that the latter can live as independent a life as possible. The starting chapter of this section is concerned with interpersonal skills and communication.

References

Berlo, D.K. (1960). *The Process of Communication: An Introduction to Theory and Practice*. New York: Holt, Rinehart and Winston.

Brammer, L.M. (1988). *The Helping Relationship; Process and Skills*. London: Allyn and Bacon.

Egan, G. (1990). *The Skilled Helper: A Systematic Approach To Effective Helping*. Pacific Grove, CA: Brooks/Cole.

Heron, J. (1970). 'The phenomenology of social encounter: The gaze.' *Philosophy and Phenomenological Research*, **31**, 243–264.

Johnson, D.W. and Johnson, F.P. (1991). *Joining Together: Group Theory and Group Skills*. Englewood Cliffs, NJ: Prentice-Hall.

Laswell, H.D. (1960). 'The structure and function of communication in society.' In: Scharamm, W. (Ed.) *Mass Communication*. Urbana, IL: University of Illinois Press.

Ley, P. (1988). *Communicating With Patients: Improving Communication, Satisfaction and Compliance*. Cambridge: Chapman and Hall.

Shannon, C.E. and Weaver, W. (1949). *The Mathematical Theory of Communication*. Urbana, IL: University of Illinois Press.

The dimensions of communication 16

Objectives

After reading this chapter you should be able to:

1 Recognise the nature and complexity of communication
2 Identify those interpersonal skills
3 Explain the mechanism of communication
4 Describe some of the 'how' and 'why' of communication
  For example:
  a Proxemics and territoriality
  b Meaning and aspects of gaze
  c Gaze as a regulator of communication
  d Effect of gaze on individuals
  e Explain and differentiate between posture and gesture
  f The use of touch
  g Aspects of touch
  h Explain paralanguage and its component
  i Explain the functions of silence in communication

Why do we communicate?

The whole purpose of communication, as Stanton (1986) says, is to be heard or received, to be understood, and to be accepted. People communicate to socialise, to express their needs, their wants, and to ventilate their feelings. People also communicate to get action, that is to influence others to behave in a certain way. This can be observed in the behaviour of politicians, especially when they are desperate for votes. From a clinical perspective however, the helper communicates to reassure patients or clients by giving them information regarding their illnesses in terms of their diagnosis, alleviating their fears and anxieties by keeping them up to date with what is going on and answer any queries they may have.

How do we communicate?

There are a variety of ways of communicating and these fall broadly into two main categories. These are

- verbal and
- non-verbal

Verbal communication

Non-verbal communication

Verbal forms of communication would include all those means which have speech and language as their foundations. Non-verbal communication however, may not be as straightforward to define. Knapp's (1978, p.3) argument suggests that it is rather difficult to dissect human interaction into two separate diagnoses, (i.e.) verbal and non-verbal. 'The verbal dimension is so intimately woven and so subtly represented in so much of what we have previously labelled non-verbal that the term does not always adequately describe the behaviour under study.' Dance (1967) believes that an individual may send information through non-vocal or non-verbal means, the receiver however may still have to use the symbols of language to decipher its meaning. In its true sense therefore, non-verbal communication may be a misnomer. Dance's (1967, p.290) point is succinctly put in the following quote, 'A verbal symbol can be either vocal or non-vocal. A vocal sound need not always be symbolic. A scream, for instance, may be vocal and non-verbal on the reflex discharge level. On the other hand, a scream, when interpreted by a passer-by in terms of circumstances, may be vocal and also may have meaning for the passer-by beyond the meaning to the screamer. Thus, the passer-by's meaning, being the result of his past actual or vicarious experience, is interpreted by him in terms of words and becomes both vocal and verbal.' For the sake of simplicity, let us assume that if those strategies adopted by the sender do not constitute any vocal or verbal means, they fall into the category of non-verbal communication. Have a go at Exercise 63.

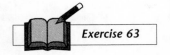

Exercise 63

Make a list of all those possible non-verbal means of communication that you can think of.

Your list may include such aspects as proxemics, posture, gesture (movement), gaze direction (eye contact and orientation), touch, facial expression, head-nods, appearance, silence and other body languages, all of which, according to Raffler-Engle (1980) are generally grouped into kinesics. The intention here is to explore some of the so-called non-verbal communication in more detail.

Proxemics and territoriality

Hall (1966, p.1) introduced the term 'proxemics' to suggest, 'interrelated observations and theories of man's use of space as a specialised elaboration of culture'. Knapp (1978) said that the term territoriality has been used for many years in the study of animal and fowl behaviour and these behaviours suggest that these animals identify with an area and will defend it against any other animals which invade it. There are three types of territories and these are primary, secondary and public.

1   Primary. This would include one's home and personal belongings.

2 Secondary. This consists of one's television set or even one's eating
   utensils. 'We are apt to see more frequent conflicts develop over
   these territories because the public/private boundary is blurred'
   (Knapp, 1978, p.116).
3 Public. This is available to all of us for a temporary period of time
   and includes such things as parks, beaches and seats on public
   transport.

Proxemics are similar to territoriality and can be described as the study
of space between people during an interaction, having said that, other factors such as gaze, touch and other body languages are significant to the
concept. These factors will be discussed separately. From Hall's (1963,
p.1003) perspective this space includes man's 'organisation of space in his
houses and buildings and ultimately the layout of his towns'. There are
three kinds of spatial organisation and these are fixed, semi-fixed feature
and informal space.

Fixed feature involves the spatial arrangement of one's environment   ***Fixed feature***
and one's house would be an example. An individual becomes extremely
distressed if his or her fixed space is intruded upon and in fact some people would refuse to live in the same house once it had been burgled.

Semi-fixed feature refers to all those moveable objects like tables, chairs   ***Semi-fixed feature***
and even cars. People become uncomfortable when others drive too near
to their vehicles.

Informal space relates to the distance between person to person in the   ***Informal space***
proper sense, for example if I was to interact with you, then our informal
space would be the distance between you and me, how near or far you are
from me.

The focus here is on the third kind of spatial organisation, that is, informal space. This is often referred to as interpersonal distance and its significance is not just so that people can hear each other better, informal space
has far greater implications than that. Danziger (1976, p.59) states that
when people talk to each other the distance they create between themselves varies very little. 'The usual nose-to-nose distance in ordinary conversation is four to five feet and variations of more than some inches either
way soon lead to feelings of discomfort.' Try the Exercise 64.

Find a colleague (not an intimate partner) and stand as close to him or her
as you physically can. Make a mental note of the degree of discomfort you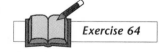
feel. Now, try and gradually create some distance between the two of you

Exercise 64

and stop whenever you feel comfortable with the distance between yourselves.

The distance which you have created between yourselves is what can be
described as your personal space and this is a significant factor in non-verbal communication. Hall (1966) identified four distance zones and these
are intimate, personal, social and public distance.

Intimate (close phase) is seen as the closest (body contact) one could   ***Intimate distance***
ever get to another person and as the name suggests, it involves people
who are intimate with one another, for example lovers and parents. Hall

called this the distance of love making, where one's sense of smell and touch are at their maximum and where verbal output is kept to a minimum. Within the intimate zone, a distance of 6 to 18 inches is considered as a far phase. Hall (1966, p.111) remarked that the, 'heads, thighs, and pelvis are not easily brought into contact but hand can reach and grasp extremities'.

Personal distance

Personal distance can range from a distance of: 1.5 to 2.5 feet, which is seen as the close phase and 2.5 to 4 feet as the far phase. Here although there is no physical contact, if so desired people involved can actually reach out and make body contact in the close phase. In the far phase of the personal distance, this may be an indication that physical contact is not intended.

Social distance

Social distance can range from a distance of: 4 to 7 feet in the near phase and 7 to 12 feet in the far phase. The belief here is that 'most impersonal informal business occurs at the closer of these distances, where the taller of the two interactants can look down at the other (such as a businessman at his secretary)' (Harper et al., 1978, p.248).

Public distance

Public distance ranges from 12 to 20 feet or more and as the name suggests there may not be a need to recognise and acknowledge people. Here there is basically much more room to manoeuvre one's movement to suit oneself. Voice and facial definitions are lost leaving the focus to be on gestures and body stance.

Hall (1968, p.84) made the point that his findings are relevant only to Americans and as such cannot be generalised to other cultural groups. 'What crowds one person does not necessarily crowd another.'

Individual differences in proxemics

The general consensus seems to be that there are in fact individual differences in the interpersonal distance and some of these differences include gender, age, culture and ethnicity, and status.

Proxemics and gender differences

According to Lett et al. (1969), females tend to maintain closer interpersonal distances than males. Hartnett et al. (1970) concluded that females in fact allow the experimenter to get closer to them than males. The gender difference of the other interactant is also significant in interpersonal distance, for example Liebman (1970) found that females tended to sit closer to other females than other males. The possible explanation rests in the fact that society seems to accept closer female to female than male to male interactions.

Proxemics and age differences

Research suggests that there is a significant difference in interpersonal distances between people of various ages. According to Meisels and Guardo (1969), children seem to require less interpersonal space as they grow older. Dennis and Powell (1972) however, concluded that older children create a greater distance between peers and teachers during interaction.

Proxemics and culture

The overall impression seems to indicate that there are differences in personal distance space between people of different cultures. For example Hall (1966) stated that Germans require more interpersonal space than Americans, French and Arabs.

Lott and Sommer (1967) cited in Danziger (1976), reported that people of equal status tend to sit closer together than people of unequal status. 'Where a status differential exists there is lack of reciprocity in the permissible closeness of approach to the other person. The lower-status individual may allow the higher-status individual to approach closely but not dare to approach such a high-status person to the same degree of closeness' (Danziger, 1976, p.60).

Proxemics and status

It could be argued that the setting of an interaction is also important in maintaining personal distance between interactants, for example interpersonal distance between two people will be less in the street than in one's home. Similarly one would stand closer to others in a queue than one would in any other place.

Proxemics and settings

Invasion and defence of our territory

Knapp (1978) stated that police interrogators are sometimes given instructions to sit very close to the suspect, without a desk in between so as not to provide any protection or comfort. This renders the suspect vulnerable and the interrogators therefore are seen as having a psychological advantage. The purpose of a desk in a classroom is not just to have something to write on, but it also provides some sort of psychological comfort, hence students' preferences for desks. Although an individual's favourite interpersonal distance is most treasured, sometimes he or she has no choice but to let it be intruded upon, even if these distances are informal or personal. Such settings as being in a lift, on a crowded bus, in a compact queue, or at a pop concert, are examples of personal space invasion. Here however the individual feels it is quite appropriate and he or she does not take offence. Similarly in a clinical setting, patients' intimate and personal zones are legitimately intruded upon in health care situations such as, the radiographer actually holding patients in front of the X-ray machine, the nurse handling and moving patients, or doctors physically examining patients. These situations suggest that the patients are at the mercy of helpers and as such are not in a position to be able to do anything. As a professional caregiver one is perceived to have the 'right' to invade the personal space of patients or clients, because of the position the professional caregivers hold in society. This is basically seen as 'we are doing it for the good of our patients'. As a health care professional therefore one needs to reflect on how it feels when someone moves in too close to oneself and with this in mind if I move too close to my patient's personal space and he or she takes a step back, this should be a clear indication that I am in fact intruding in his or her personal space. What I should then do is to ensure that this distance is kept, instead of keep on entering his or her personal space. Some types of territorial encroachments are seen as acceptable, other types of encroachment are frowned upon, for example how do you feel when someone occupies your seat? How do you feel, if someone comes and sits next to you on an empty bus? If there is no justifying reasons for the encroachment of one's territory, then one would feel uncomfortable and perhaps even angry. According to Lyman and Scott (1967) there are three types of territorial encroachments and these are violation, invasion and contamination.

Violation

Violation is described as the unwarranted use of another person's territory and this could include such behaviour as, staring at people whilst they are eating in a restaurant, and making too much noise.

Invasion

Invasion feels more like a permanent thing, as when a country is invaded. Invasion is also reflected when one basically takes over a room, for example I could turn my kitchen into a study by spreading books all over the place and working there all the time.

Contamination

Contamination occurs when, for example, an individual goes and stays at a friend's place and he or she leaves things, like a dirty shirt or a similar item, behind after the stay. Similarly when people stay in a hotel, they are displeased if they find things which belonged to the previous occupier. Contamination is also related to deeds such as other people's dogs littering one's garden.

According to Knapp the two primary methods of defence are prevention and reaction.

Prevention

Prevention is akin to marking one's territory so that other people will recognise it and move elsewhere, like the classic British joke of the Germans and their towels. Sometimes an item of clothing is used to stake out a seat so that people know that it is occupied. Alternatively people may ask someone else to look after their seats.

Reaction

Reaction is related to the way one reacts and this depends on how the intrusion is perceived, for example if I perceive the intrusion as positive then I will reciprocate and if I interpret the intrusion as negative, then according to Knapp, I may adopt anyone of the following behaviours: looking away; changing the topic to a less personal one; crossing my arms to form a frontal barrier to the invasion; covering certain parts of my body; rubbing my neck and in the process my elbow will protrude toward the invader. People can also display both defensive and offensive reactions.

Gaze

An overall definition of gaze is that it is an individual's visual or looking behaviour. According to Cranach (1971), there are various types of looking behaviour and these include:

- One-sided gaze, which is simply defined as a person looking at another person's face
- Face gaze is the directing of one person's face at another person's face
- Eye gaze is directing one person's gaze at another person's eyes
- Mutual gaze is where two interactants look at each other in the face
- Eye contact is where one person specifically looks at the other person's eyes and in this sense both are aware of the gaze of the other
- Gaze avoidance is the avoidance of another person's eye gaze

Eyes have been referred to as the windows of the soul. Many messages are sent and received by the eyes. Such statements like, 'Your eyes say it all,' 'Don't look at me that way,' 'Look at me when I am talking to you,' 'There is sadness in your eyes,' 'You give me that confused look,' and 'Come on' eyes, are perhaps an indication of the different messages that the eyes convey. According to Danziger (1976), people have communicated by means of the eyes since ancient times, through the concept of 'The Evil Eye'. As Heron (1970) said, the true concept of meeting another person is when both people actually look at each other in their eyes. It is still unclear, however, as to what constitutes normal gazing. How long is one supposed to look at another or better still whose eyes is one permitted to look at? The answers to some of the above questions are culturally defined. According to Myers and Myers (1992), children in Black or Hispanic cultures were brought up not to look in the face of their elders. White middle-class cultures on the other hand demand eye contact from their children.

The meaning of gaze

Where to look

People know how comfortable or uncomfortable it feels when they are being gazed at by strangers, but what exactly does gazing behaviour indicate? Argyle states that there is less gaze during deeper self-disclosures. There is no doubt that gaze tells its own story. Society's norm allows people to look at one another as long as they restrict themselves to certain specific areas of the body, for example it is quite acceptable to look at people above the neck but if we are to look at other specific regions such as the breasts, pelvis, and legs, our motives are questionable. A man looking at a woman's breast region, or a woman looking at a man's genital area, could be interpreted as sexual advances. Having said that, this could also be seen as invasion of personal space. 'His eyes give me the creeps,' reflects this sentiment. Gazing is also conditional on one's likes or dislikes. If a person shows more gaze during an interaction, he or she is likely to be seen as attentive. Similarly less gaze on the part of the listener is perceived as passive and inattentive.

According to Argyle (1988), the basic statistics for two people in conversation on a neutral kind of topic and at a distance of 6 feet are as represented in Table 16.1.

How long to look

Table 16.1
Source Argyle (1988) *Bodily Communication*, Routledge

Individual gaze	60%
While listening	75%
While talking	40%
Length of glance	3 seconds
Eye-contact	30%
Length of mutual glance	1.5 seconds

There is less gaze at closer distances than at long distances.

Gaze can be seen as both a sign of intimacy, when you look at your partner's eyes, and as showing one's disapproval to others, as in the case of Lionel Blair when he was heckled, in one of Noel Edmond's television pranks (The House Party). The Blair stare was ferocious. Argyle says that glances are timed to collect information and when needed, people will

Why do we look

look, when not needed people tend to look away. When there is something different, perhaps a facially disfigured person, there is an element of prolongation of gaze. This is particularly so if the gazer thinks he or she can get away with it. Try Exercise 65.

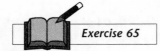

Exercise 65

Make a list of the people you have a tendency to look or stare at.

Your list may have included any group of people who are different to yourself, such as:

- Disfigured people
- Pregnant women
- Physically attractive people
- Physically unattractive people
- Black and other ethnic minorities
- Non-conformists
- Fat and slim people
- Behavioural abnormality
- Celebrities

According to Kendon (1967), there are four functions of gazing and these are to:

1   Regulate the flow of communication
2   Monitor feedback
3   Express emotion
4   Communicate the nature of interpersonal relationships

Regulate communication

In regulating the flow of communication the eyes alone can sometimes indicate that one has the desire to engage in conversation. I can recall numerous occasions when I could not remember the name of my students, all I had to do was to look at them and they would respond. Many students try frequently to avoid eye contact with their teachers in an attempt to avoid being asked questions, and as Knapp (1978) said, the last thing you want to do is to give the impression that your channels of communication are open. Knapp also pointed out that in a restaurant, all one has to do to attract the attention of the waiter is to just look at them or in their direction and they will respond. Similarly some of us will be familiar with the way we go about avoiding eye contact with those collecting for charities in an attempt to escape feeling embarrassed. In terms of regulating the flow of communication, Knapp (1978, p.298) has this to say, 'eye behaviour also regulates the flow of communication by providing turn-taking signals. . . . The speaker–listener pattern seems to be choreographed as follows: As the speaker comes to the end of an utterance or thought unit, gazing at the listener will continue as the listener assumes the speaking role; the listener will maintain gaze until the speaking role is assumed when he or she will look away.'

Monitor feedback

Knapp stated that when people seek feedback concerning the reactions of others, they gaze at them. Similarly if people look at us when we speak, it is usually a sign that they are interested in what we are talking about.

According to Ekman and Friesen (1975) various emotions can be detected from one's face.

Express emotion

When eyebrows are raised so that they are curved and high, it indicates surprise; the eyebrows raised and drawn together show fear; lowering the brows and upper eyelids mean disgust; brows are lowered and drawn together to suggest anger; the bottom eyelids show wrinkles and may be raised to show happiness; the inner corners of the eyebrows are drawn up and the skin below the brow is triangulated, indicating sadness.

The effects of emotion on gaze

The common belief in communicating the nature of interpersonal relationships is that people tend to look more at people they like and less at people they dislike. Danziger (1976, p.64) states that in interview situations, if the interviewer is more positive toward the interviewee, the latter will show more eye contact. Similarly induction of negative affect leads to less eye contact. If I was to ask you a personal or an embarrassing question it is most likely that you will avoid eye contact. Many times when we have done something embarrassing we say things like 'I didn't know where to put my face'. Burying our face in our hands is also a common gesture.

Communicate the nature of interpersonal relationships

What can an individual do when he or she is being gazed at? There are in fact two options, (1) he or she can look back or (2) he or she can look away.

Imagine that three people are involved in a conversation, but only two of them are engaged in mutual gaze, the third person will feel left out and sooner or later he or she will cease to take part in the conversation. How would you feel if the lecturer looked only at one student in the classroom? You would probably think that he or she has a liking for that particular student and you would probably be correct. The effects of gaze on people can be viewed from two perspectives, these are positive and negative. Some of the positive effects of being looked at include: a feeling that people are interested in the individual, the one who is gazing may be interested in initiating some sort of interaction with an individual (Argyle, 1988). Some of the negative effects of gaze are:

Effects of gaze on us

- a feeling of discomfort
- self-doubt
- becoming angry
- wondering why
- becoming self-conscious
- feeling threatened
- becoming paranoid

According to Knapp, the following situations are likely to lead to more gazing:

Situations where more gazing is predicted

- when one is physically distant from the other person
- when the topics are easy and impersonal
- when there is nothing else to look at
- when an individual is interested in the reactions of another person
- when one is of a lower status than the other person

- when an individual is trying to dominate or influence another person
- if this is part of one's culture
- extrovert
- when one wants to be involved or included in say, a discussion
- when an individual is listening as compared to talking
- when the person is a female

Situations where less gazing is predicted

Some of the situations where less gaze is predicted include the following:

- when one is physically close
- when one is engaged in difficult or intimate topics
- when there are many other things to look at
- when one is not interested in the other person's reaction
- when one is talking as compared to listening
- if an individual dislikes the other person
- in a scenario of I'm OK but you're not OK
- cultural prohibition
- when one does not need or want to be involved
- in some mental health problems (i.e.) depression
- an introvert

Posture and gesture

It would be true to say that the most communication is achieved without speaking and this is reflected in Freud's sentiments, as quoted by Ekman and Friesen (1969, p.89), 'he that has eyes to see and ears to hear and may convince himself that no mortal can keep a secret. If his lips are silent, he chatters with his finger-tips; betrayal oozes out of him at every pore.' If the eyes do not give the game away, the face will, and if the face does not, the body certainly will, and this will be in the form of gesture and posture. One basically cannot escape from revealing oneself to the world in one way or another. You can still be heard even if no sound comes out of your mouth, your very existence will speak its own language.

Gesture

Thumbs up, you live and thumbs down you die, such was the power of gesture in ancient Rome. Lamb and Watson (1979) define gesture as any movement which is confined to one or more parts of the body, like Churchill's classic V-sign to imply victory, parents' pointing finger to suggest that they are not happy with their children's behaviour, or the rude one or two finger sign to ask someone to go away.

Posture

Posture on the other hand is defined as movements which involved the whole of the body. Having said that, gesture needs to be congruent with posture for the message to be clear. As Lamb and Watson (1979, p.11)

The false smile

said, a cheery wave needs to be congruent with an uplifted posture and not with a slumped posture. 'Because most of us are quite good at detecting this degree of discrepancy between a gesture and its expected meaning, and can recognise the smile that is "for real," those who think their job requires a battery of smiles, or grew up to believe that "the whole world loves a smile," might come on better without their grins.' The superficial gesture of a salesperson is designed to lull people into a false sense of security, it is not designed as an initiator of a long-lasting relationship. Having said that it is very difficult to make sense of a smiling gesture on its own. One could argue that gestures can only be read in relation to the whole of the body posture and only then can one make sense of what is going on.

According to Bull (1987), there have been many claims for the psychological significance of posture, for example one can obtain valuable information about a person's emotions and attitudes, social relationships, and the structure of the social interaction. Posture can also be seen as a therapeutic tool, although there is not much evidence to support this. Personal experience suggests that this may be true. Gesture, especially hands or head movements, more often accompany speaking.

Posture and emotion

Most of the evidence seems to suggest that the face is the most effective channel for communicating emotion, but according to Argyle (1988), certain specific emotions are communicated better through body movement. Anger would be one such emotion, 'a tense person sits or stands rigidly, upright or leaning forwards, often with hands clasped together, legs together, muscles tense. . . . . Depressives have a drooping, listless posture, and sit brooding, looking at the floor. Manics are alert and erect, their body in a high degree of arousal' (Argyle, 1988, p.210).

According to Mehrabian (1968), if I am to lean forward towards you during an interaction, this would be indicative of a positive attitude, as compared to a backward lean, which conveys a negative attitude. Posture can also convey certain aspects of one's personality. Argyle (1988) said that posture is probably affected by body image, for example adolescent girls who are proud of their breasts will adopt quite different postures in comparison to those who are ashamed of their breasts. Similarly people may either display or conceal their height, their legs, or other features of their bodies depending on their attitudes and feelings towards these.

Touch

The study of how touch is used in communication is called haptics. Touch is probably one of the most revealing and most important means of all non-verbal communication. A clinician holding the hand of a patient will generate an element of warmth in his or her behaviour, a handshake will indicate a social relationship in the form of a greeting, a kiss will suggest intimacy, a hug may be interpreted as a gesture of comfort and security, and a punch, a smack or a kick, well you know what it means. As was discussed in Chapter 3, touch has both biological and psychological implications and perhaps it would be correct to assume that without touch people would be deprived of one of the most basic of human needs. This could have serious consequences for their growth and development. Some would say that touching, in fact, influences disclosure and compliance (Tubbs and Moss, 1994). In common everyday language many terms are used to signify the importance of touch in one's interaction. Montagu's (1978) list of such terms includes:

- rubbing people the wrong way
- stroking
- soft touch
- thick-skinned
- get in touch
- handling people carefully
- making contact
- getting under my skin
- skin-deep
- touchy

According to Jones and Yarbrough (1985), some of the different types of touches are:

- positive affect and this would include the showing of affection, appreciation, inclusion (and this may be when we physically grab hold of someone to get him or her to come with us), and sexual touches
- ritualistic, consists of all those touches with which one is involved as a matter of routine, like in greeting and farewell
- task-related, as when in working close to someone else, for instance nursing, physiotherapy, radiography, radiotherapy, dentistry and medicine, where touch is one of the most important mediums for support and communication
- playful, which is when one is having fun
- control, which is apparent in compliance behaviour, for example physically holding someone to prevent injury to self and others
- accidental, which is usually followed by an apology

Heslin's (1974) classification of touching behaviour, on the other hand, has five categories which are based on the nature of the interpersonal relationship and these are:

1   Functional or professional level
2   Social or polite level
3   Friendship or warmth level
4   Love or intimacy level
5   Sexual arousal level

Professional level of touch

Functional or professional level, here the use of touch is more on an impersonal level, like a professional caregiver and his or her patient. Knapp (1978) described this as businesslike touching where the other person is seen as an object or non-person. This is the caregiver's way of keeping any intimate or sexual messages from interfering with the task at hand.

The social or polite level includes the touch which is involved in hand- *Social level*
shakes. Physical contact which occurs is confined to a socially prescribed
level and the purpose is to acknowledge the existence of the other person.

Friendship or warmth level. Harper *et al.* (1978) said that this level is *Friendship level*
most difficult for people to interpret because of its closeness to love or sexual attraction, thus when two friends are alone, this type of touching will
decrease because privacy is linked or associated with sex and love.

Love or intimacy level. The aim here is to show one's feeling and inten- *Intimacy level*
tion to the other person. As Knapp said, when we lay our hands on the
cheeks of a person or when we are kissing the other person, we are basically expressing an emotional attachment or attraction through touch.

Sexual arousal level. This is probably the most intense of all the levels *Sexual arousal level*
of touch and the aim here is sexually orientated. Your imagination is
called for here.

The two faces of touch: warmth and dominance

Argyle states that touch has two main dimensions of meaning and these
are warmth and dominance. One could say that most of the professional
type of touches would be classified under the warmth touch and all those
which involve aggression and violence could be seen as some form of dominance touch. Argyle's (1988, p.227) vocabulary of touch simplifies this
point (see Table 16.2).

Therapeutic touch

Generally speaking any use of touch which enhances growth and development on the part of the client can be seen as therapeutic. This would
seem to fit in with Heslin's functional or professional level of touch.
Personal experience suggests that the use of touch makes a qualitative difference in terms of caring, it brings a human element to the role of a
helper. In a study conducted by Aguilera (1967), psychiatric nurses
employed simple but appropriate touch gestures whilst verbally interacting with their patients and the result showed more verbal interaction on
the part of the patients after approximately 8 days of interaction. Having
said that, it has to be stressed that therapeutic touch, as with some other
non-verbal communication, is culturally defined. This suggests that touch
may be therapeutic in one culture and non-therapeutic in another culture.
This therefore has serious implications for care delivery.

Paralanguage

The discussion thus far has been on the non-verbal aspects of communication. Having said that, many communication theorists would agree that
the ways or means of communication is never neutral. One does not just
communicate at any particular time in either verbal or non-verbal. In fact

it would be true to say that people use a mixture of channels to communicate their messages. The channels of communication consist of more than just verbal and non-verbal. One other aspect of communication is that of paralanguage. Paralanguage can be described as a hybrid (mixture) between verbal and non-verbal communication. Some would describe paralanguage as the vocal cues which accompany spoken words and as such are seen as content free. Paralanguage emphasises the 'how' of what is being said.

Table 16.2
Argyle's vocabulary of touch. Argyle (1988) *Bodily Communication*

Touch	Meaning
Stroke, caress, lick: body, face, hair	Sex, affection
Pat: hand, arm, back	Friendship, reassurance, support
Shake hand, formal kiss, hug, embrace	Greeting, parting
Sustained embrace, hand-holding	Enjoy close relationships
Touch hand, arm, or shoulder while speaking	Enhancing social influence
Brief touch	Getting attention
Pull, push, guide	Direct movement
Professional touches, e.g. medical	Attending to the body, but non-social
Tickle	Play
Hit, scratch, slap, kick	Aggression

Components of paralanguage

According to Trager (1958), the components of paralanguage include:

- Voice qualities: these consist of pitch range, vocal lip control, articulation control, rhythm control, resonance, and tempo.
- Vocal characterisers: these relate to elements like laughing, crying, whispering, snoring, yelling, moaning, groaning, yawning, whining, stretching, sucking, spitting, sneezing, coughing, clearing of the throat, sniffing, sighing, swallowing, heavily marked inhaling or exhaling, belching, and hiccuping.
- Vocal qualifiers: these include intensity, and pitch height.
- Vocal segregates: these are the uh, um, uh-huh, and silent pauses.

Danziger (1976, p.70) said that it is clear, certain paralinguistic signs increase the impact of verbal messages. 'Intonation is of course also used to regulate the alternation of listening and speaking in conversation. But beyond this the role of non-verbal speech qualities in social interaction remains largely a matter of everyday impressions and speculation.'

Silence

It is said that silence can only be defined in general and its meaning has to be seen in the context in which it occurs. Silence can be described as a pause between speech and it can be taken to mean anything from not wanting to say anything to not knowing what to say. Myers and Myers (1992) highlight a list of 11 different meanings associated with silence. Some of these include:

1   When one is angry and frustrated but refuses to let off steam
2   When one is attentively listening to something important
3   When one is bored
4   When one cannot think of what to say
5   When one is thinking about what the speaker has said
6   When one does not understand what the speaker has said
7   When scenery is so beautiful that it makes an individual speechless (as in taking your breath away)

The following could be added to this list.

When one feels there's no more to be said on the matter
When an individual is very much in love and all he or she wants to do is to hold the other in silence
When one is in grief
When teacher asks at the end of lesson, 'any questions?'

This list can no doubt be extended, however the main focus is on the therapeutic use of silence and this is discussed in Chapter 17, where the concept of listening, attending and responding are explored.

References

Aguilera, D.C. (1967). 'Relationships between physical contact and verbal interaction between nurses and patients.' *Journal of Psychiatric Nursing* 5, 5–21.

Argyle, M. (1988). *Bodily Communication*. London: Routledge.

Bull, P. (1987). *Body Movement and Interpersonal Communication*. Chichester, New York: John Wiley and Sons.

Cranach, M. (1971). 'The role of orienting behaviour in human interaction.' In: Esser, A.H. (Ed.) *Behaviour and Environment: The Use of Space by Animals and Men*. New York: Plenum Press, pp. 217–237.

Dance, F.E.X. (1967). *Toward a Theory of Human Communication, Human Communication Theory*. New York: Holt, Rinehart and Winston.

Danziger, K. (1976). *Interpersonal Communication*. Oxford: Pergamon Press.

Dennis, V.C. and Powell, E.R. (1972). 'Non-verbal communication.' In: *Across-Race Dyads. Summary of Proceedings of the 80th Annual Convention of the American Psychological Association*. Washington, DC: American Psychological Association, pp. 557–558.

Ekman, P. and Friesen, W.V. (1969). 'Non verbal leakage and clues to decephon.' *Psychiatry*, **32**, 88–105.

Ekman, P. and Friesen, W.V. (1975). *Unmasking the Face.* Englewood Cliffs, NJ: Prentice-Hall.

Hall, E.T. (1963). 'A system for the notation of proxemic behaviour.' *American Anthropologist*, **65**, 1003–1026.

Hall, E.T. (1966). *The Hidden Dimension.* Garden City, New York: Doubleday.

Hall, E.T. (1968). 'Proxemics.' *Current Anthropology*, **9**, 83–108.

Harper, R.G., Wiens, A.N. and Matarazzo, J.D. (1978). *Non-verbal Communication. The State of the Art.* Chichester: John Wiley and Sons.

Hartnett, J.J., Bailey, K.G. and Gibson, F.W. Jr. (1970). 'Personal space as influenced by sex and type of movement.' *Journal of Psychology*, **76**, 139–144.

Heron, J. (1990). *Helping The Client: A Creative Practical Guide.* London: Sage.

Heslin, R. (1974). 'Steps toward a taxonomy of touching.' Paper presented at the meeting of the Western Psychological Association, Chicago.

Jones, S.E. and Yarbrough, E. (1985). 'A naturalistic study of the meanings of touch.' *Communication Monographs*, **52**, 19–56.

Kendon, A. (1967). 'Some functions of gaze-direction in social interaction.' *Acta Psychologica*, **26**, 22–63.

Knapp, M.L. (1978). *Non-Verbal Communication in Human Interaction.* London: Holt, Rinehart and Winston.

Lamb, W. and Watson, E. (1979). *Body Code; The Meaning in Movement.* London: Routledge and Kegan Paul.

Lett, E.E., Clark, W. and Altman, I. (1969). 'A propositional inventory on research on interpersonal distance.' Research Report No.1, Bethesda: Naval Medical Research Institute.

Liebman, M. (1970). 'The effects of sex and race norms on personal space.' *Environment and Behaviour*, **2**, 208–246.

Lott, D.F. and Sommer, R. (1967). 'Seating arrangement and status.' *Journal of Personality and Social Psychology*, **7**, 90–95.

Lyman, S.M. and Scott, M.B. (1967). 'Territoriality: A neglected sociological dimension.' *Social Problems*, **15**, 235–249.

Mehrabian, A. (1968). 'Inference of attitudes from the posture, orientation and distance of a communicator.' *Journal of Consulting and Clinical Psychology*, **32**, 296–308.

Meisels, M. and Guardo, C.J. (1969). 'Development of personal space schemas.' *Child Development*, **40**, 1167–1178.

Montagu, A. (1978). *Touching: The Human Significance of the Skin.* New York: Harper and Row.

Myers, G.E. and Myers, M.T. (1992). *The Dynamics of Human Communication: A Laboratory Approach.* London: McGraw-Hill.

Rafler-Engle, W. (1980). *Aspects of Non-Verbal Communication.* Swets and Zeitlinger B.V.-Lisse.

Stanton, N. (1986). *The Business of Communicating: Improving Your Communication Skills.* London and Sydney: Pan Books.

Trager, G.L. (1958). 'Paralanguage: A first approximation.' *Studies in Linguistics,* **13**, 1–12.

Tubbs, S. L. and Moss, S. (1994). *Human Communication.* London: McGraw-Hill.

Listening, attending and responding 17

Objectives

After reading this chapter you should be able to:

1   Define listening, attending and responding
2   Differentiate between listening and hearing
3   List and explain some of the types of listening
4   Explain the 'why' of listening
5   Describe some of the barriers to therapeutic listening
6   Identify and explain some appropriate ways of responding
7   Explain the relationship between communication and standard of care delivery

Listening, attending and responding, the elements of a therapeutic relationship

The foundation for a therapeutic relationship is based on the concepts of listening, attending and responding. The dynamic relationships between these terms are such that there is an element of interdependency amongst them. If for example I am unable to give my fullest attention to you, it is most likely that I would miss most of what you tell me and my response to you may be totally inappropriate. The correct recipe is to fully attend, listen and then respond. Listening can be defined as the art of capturing the true essence of the sender's message. Art is taken to mean skill and ability. The word 'capturing' is used deliberately because of its implication of being an active process, which the listener has to engage in. According to Barker (1971), the process of listening involves four different, yet, interrelated processes and these are:

1   Attending
2   Hearing
3   Understanding
4   Remembering

Attending

Attending is the art of being both physically (with exceptions) and psychologically present and in tune with what is being said. Although this may come across as simple and easy to engage in, it is extremely difficult to practice. Do you ever recall a time when someone was talking to you and all of a sudden you had a thought in your head which was totally unconnected with what the other person was saying? If this was the case then one would say you were not truly in an attentive mode to this other person. The argument would be that whilst this intruding thought was gaining access to your concentration, your attention would have been diluted by it and this would mean not being in a position to capture the whole of the speaker's sentiment. Transfer this concept into a carer–client scenario and one could imagine how a client's message can be misheard, misunderstood and therefore forgotten and the resulting response would be negative. Response in this context is taken to mean the giving of appropriate feedback to the message received.

Rankin (1926), cited in Myers and Myers (1992), conducted a study to find out what percentage of people's time is spent listening. He asked his subjects to record at 15-minute intervals, during their waking day, the length of time they spent in four different types (listening, talking, reading, and writing) of communication. Rankin's report showed that 70 per cent of his subjects' waking day were spent in one or more of these kinds of communication. A detailed breakdown of the result is shown in Table 17.1.

How much of our time is spent listening?

Table 17.1
A breakdown of the percentages of communication based on 70 per cent of Rankin's subjects' waking day

Type of communication	Percentage
Listening	45%
Talking	30%
Reading	16%
Writing	9%

Rankin's conclusion was that, listening is the form of communication most frequently employed during an average waking day. Numerous other studies have supported Rankin's claim. This would suggest that listening is indeed a very important aspect of communication.

Listening is not the same as hearing

It would be an understatement to say that listening and hearing are two distinct processes. Say for example I gave a lecture which lasted for 1 hour. Although most of the audience, if not all, would hear me speaking, it may well be that only a few of them were actually listening. Listening by definition is not a natural process, it means paying attention, remembering and understanding the speaker's speech content. Hearing on the other hand is a natural process, which suggests that one does not have to learn to hear. Similarly it could be said that one does not have any control of what one hears. If the sound is in the waves then it is destined for your ears. As Adler and Rodman (1982, p.90) said, 'Barring illness, injury, or earplugs, hearing cannot be stopped. Your ears will pick up sound waves and transmit them to your brain whether you want them or not.'

Types of listening

There are numerous types of listening, these may not all be therapeutic. Some of these types of listening are highlighted by Barker (1971) and they include:

- Selective listening, which is listening to certain aspects of the message. This could be intentional or unintentional.
- Concentrated listening is listening to the whole message. There is an attempt to understand the whole of what the other person is saying.
- Appreciative listening leads one to recognise the tone and mood of the speaker. It also means deriving a sense of pleasure out of the whole experience, like in listening to a piece of music.
- Conversational listening is a two way kind of listening where there is a transaction between two speakers. The speaker and listener's roles are interchangeable, where one is the speaker while the other is the listener and vice versa.
- Courteous listening has a therapeutic element, for example when listening to, say, a friend, who wants to vent his or her feelings. Similarly people may want to use friends or colleagues as sounding boards.
- Listening to indicate love or respect like in the interaction between parents and their children. Children like to be listened to and when this is absent, they feel neglected.
- Critical listening is listening with a critical ear, the sole purpose of which is to make critical judgement about what has been said.
- Discriminative listening is listening for the purpose of understanding and remembering. Discriminative listening consists of four types of listening.

    1 Attentive listening, which suggests paying attention to what is being said.
    2 Retentive listening, which involves an element of understanding and remembering.
    3 Reflective listening consists not only of understanding and remembering the message, but also an evaluative aspect of what has been said and bringing this to the fore.
    4 Reactive listening involves responding to the speaker. Here the listener is attentive and reflective, and then offers a response to the speaker.

Why do we listen?

There are numerous reasons why one listens, these however can be broad-ly classified under two main headings, serious listening and social listen-ing. Barker (1971) said that serious listening involves listening with a spe-cific purpose to comprehend, understand, remember, evaluate, or criticise. Serious listening falls under two basic categories of rewards: general and specific. General rewards for serious listening include the following:

Reward listening

- Help to expand one's knowledge, one basically learns as one listens
- Develop command of one's language
- Evaluate strong and weak points in a message

Specific rewards for serious listening include:

- You pass your exams if you listen
- You save time and money
- You make a shortcut to knowledge (if you listen to the lecturer, you may have enough information to help you through your work)

Social listening is listening for pleasure, this would include such things as listening to radio, television, music or a pop concert. The rewards for social listening include:

Social listening

- Increasing the enjoyment of your aural stimuli
- Enlarging your experience
- Expanding your interests, awareness of cultural and ethnic influ-ences
- Improving your personality and self-confidence
- Therapeutic, which means that the listener may find it helpful in some way or other

Therapeutic listening

According to Tedeschi (1990), there are three components of therapeutic listening and these are:

- Attention to the client. This involves a face to face arrangement, which has become known as the listening microskills. Egan (1977) has in fact popularised the concept of microskills by his acronym S.O.L.E.R.
  S = Sit squarely, which can be interpreted to mean sit facing the client, this however does not necessarily mean directly opposite. As long as the helper adopts an upright sitting position, as compared to a slouching posture, the client will pick up the message of a car-ing posture.
  O = Open posture means sitting with legs and arms uncrossed. A posture which has both the arms and legs crossed is said to portray

Attention to the client

a closed position, and this would suggest an element of defensiveness on the part of the helper.

L = Lean slightly forward. One needs to add here that leaning depends very much on the flow of the conversation. It could well be that the helper may have to lean away from the client at times. Think of it this way, leaning forward without leaning away will eventually land the helper right in the intimate zone of the client. This can be very unnerving and threatening for the client.

E = Eye contact. It is recommended that eye contact is kept consistent but not as a constant stare. Fixed or constant gaze can be very uncomfortable and again threatening (see Chapter 16).

R = Relax. The helper has to be relaxed in order to instil confidence in the client of his or her knowledge and skills. Imagine being lectured by a lecturer who shows lack of confidence. What sort of an impression will this have on you? You will probably walk out at the end of the lesson with the belief that the lecturer did not know what he or she was talking about. This would parallel the feeling of the client if the latter is faced with a helper who is not relaxed. Egan said that to be relaxed is to be at home with the person. Being at home is taken to mean being comfortable and at ease. Being too relaxed however may portray an attitude of boredom.

According to Tedeschi (1990, p.39), these microskills are also important in orientating the therapist toward the client. Both 'physically and psychologically so that the therapist is in a position to hear the important elements of the client's story. . .'

Attention to the therapist's own personal experience and his reactions to the client

- Attention to the therapist's own personal experience (from an internal frame of reference) and his reactions to the client. This is very much the domain of intrapersonal dynamics. Tedeschi said that the meanings of the client's messages are most accurately and richly decoded by the therapist's unconscious ones and not the surface ones. The suggestion here is that the therapist uses self as a therapeutic tool for helping the client. As Reik (1948, p.146) said, these unconscious feelers are there to search for the problem and not to master it. 'One of the peculiarities of the third ear works in two ways. It can catch what other people do not say and it can be turned inward. It can hear voices from within the self that are otherwise not audible because they are drowned out by the noise of our conscious thought-processes.'

Use of theoretical information and similar sources of knowledge

- Use of theoretical information and similar sources of knowledge. This would make sense in many ways. Just think, how would the professional caregiver ever know that the client was playing what Berne (1964) described as a 'Yes but game', if he or she had no conception of what a 'Yes but game' is? As the carer listens to clients they can use their theoretical framework to understand what the clients are really saying. 'These therapists listen for the client statements of low self-esteem which tend to be associated with a lack of trust in one's own judgement and a rejection of the value of certain aspects of one's own perception. Such perceptions are then distorted in conscious awareness so that they conform to the client's notion of others' judgements of acceptability' (Tedeschi (1990) in McGregor and White, 1990, p.45).

Barriers to therapeutic listening

Since the suggestion is that self be used as a tool for therapeutic listening, then it needs to be acknowledged that there are certain human failings that need to be taken into account. As human beings we are bound to allow our biases to interfere with our interpretation of the client's disclosure. Some of the major barriers include:

One's thoughts
Feelings
Values
Beliefs
Attitudes
Prejudices
Inner conflicts
Likes and dislikes
Opinions and ideas
Perceptions and inferences
Past experiences and memories
Assumptions
Interpretations
One's ability to differentiate and discriminate, and
One's morals.

It could be said that the most important barrier to therapeutic listening is the helper him or herself. Other factors which can hinder therapeutic listening are the helper's lack of skills and knowledge. 'The ideal therapeutic listener would be a psychotherapist who is conversant with his own inner life and not frightened by its ambiguity of a client's unconscious messages' (Tedeschi, 1990, p.49).

Barker's (1971, p.55) list of variables which may influence listening behaviour includes:

- Listener characteristics, experiences, and abilities
- Motivation and curiosity
- Interest and attitudes
- Listener's fatigue
- Speaker's qualities
- Speaker's rate of speaking
- Who the speaker is
- How well the speaker is liked
- The message and its emotional appeal
- Environment

Other factors which are particularly relevant to therapeutic listening are:

- Viewing what the client says as unimportant or uninteresting
- Getting emotionally involved
- Factual listening which, as Barker said, in some instances can be a dangerous habit. The listener could be so involved with the facts that important messages are lost
- Preparing to answer questions whilst the speaker is still speaking
- Allowing oneself to be distracted
- Faking attention or pretending to listen. This is also known as pseudolistening
- Listening only to what is easy to understand

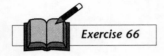

Exercise 66

Find a colleague and sit facing him or her, but as close to him or her as you physically can. I am basically asking you to intrude into the other person's intimate or personal zone. Let your colleague be the speaker (choose a fairly serious topic, this may inhibit the element of fun which will dilute the essence of the exercise) and listen to him or her for 5 minutes. Then reverse roles, you assume the speaker's role and let your colleague be the listener. After you've both had your turn at being the listener, each of you will make note of:

- what you recall in your listener's role
- all those thoughts and feelings you had during the exercise, while you were listening to your colleague
- behaviour you exhibited during the listening process

Compare notes with your colleague and discuss any emerging issues.

Proxemics and listening

Your discussion from the above exercise will lead you to conclude that the distance between you and your colleague would have contributed to your inability to listen to each other. The implication of therapeutic listening is that the clinician has to establish the appropriate distancing between himself or herself and the client, for true therapeutic listening to take place. Thoughts, feelings and behaviour similar to those which were experienced during the above exercise will interfere with the listening process. Try Exercise 67.

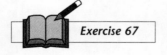

Exercise 67

Again find yourself a colleague, this time establish what you both feel is the right proxemics for a comfortable chat. This time the listener holds a constant gaze at the speaker (speaker to speak for 5 minutes). Compare notes and explore thoughts, feelings and behaviour. Discuss any emerging issues.

Gaze and listening

Exercise 67 will have introduced you to some of the difficulties experienced with unskilled gazing. As discussed previously, the listener needs to maintain consistent eye contact, but not a constant stare. The gaze has to be natural, not forced.

Other listening exercises you could try are:

1. Sit back to back with a colleague and hold a conversation, again in listener and speaker roles. Process the exercise according to the concept of experiential learning (concrete experience, observations and reflections, formation of abstract concepts and generalisations, and testing implication of concepts in new situations) which was discussed in the introduction to this book.

Exercise 68

2. A variation to the above is to sit side by side.

Exercise 69

Other issues that could be addressed are the concept of attractiveness and listening. Imagine you are listening to a most attractive (subjective) person, again in terms of thoughts, feelings and behaving, to what extent would this affect your listening ability?

Similarly, imagine you are listening to a most unattractive (again subjective) person, consider the implications for therapeutic listening.

Responding

Responding can be defined as the art of giving appropriate feedback to the message received. Obviously responding would involve the processes of listening and attending. Egan said that responding lies at the heart of the process of interpersonal communication and if one is to communicate effectively, then one has to master the skills of responding with accurate understanding. 'The ultimate proof of good listening is good responding' (Egan, 1977, p.137). Listening without responding is seen as hollow listening. Responding with understanding is the recipe for caring. Responding with understanding suggests that the listener:

*   listens carefully to the client's total message
*   recognises the speaker's feeling and the behaviour which gave rise to these feelings
*   demonstrates empathic understanding

There are numerous ways of responding to a client and these would fall under the headings of verbal, non-verbal and paralanguage.

Verbal responding

Verbal responding would include all those activities which involve making some sort of verbal statements, some of which are illustrated in the following.

Questioning. Some (Adler and Rodman, 1982) would say that questioning is a way of helping others to think about their problems, whereas oth-

Questioning

ers (Egan, 1977, in particular) see questioning as poor substitutes for responding with understanding. Questioning can be useful depending on its appropriateness in terms of context and timing. Questioning is a way of letting clients know that the helper wants to understand their situations or problems clearly. It is also a way of helping them to clarify their own situation for themselves, for example 'you said that you don't get any support at home, what would you like your wife/husband to do?' Having said that, if the questions are too selective or personal, these may lead to a non-therapeutic interaction, where the client may feel exposed and vulnerable. Adler and Rodman (1982) point to two possible dangers of inappropriate questioning and these are:

- Questioning may lead the client on a wild goose chase away from a solution to his or her problem
- Questioning can be a way of disguising advice or criticism

Open and closed questions

Most communication theorists would say that there are two types of questions which clients can be asked. These are described as open and closed questions. Open questions are those questions which encourage the client to say more about the topic, whereas closed questions lead to minimal information being offered by the client. There is a tendency to believe that the helper should always go for open question because by its very nature an open question would illicit more information from the client. This however, is not necessarily true, the nature of questioning depends on what exactly the helper wants to find out or how much information the latter wants. If all one wants to know from the client is a 'yes' or a 'no', then it is quite legitimate for the helper to ask a closed question. Similarly asking the patient his or her name could be interpreted as a closed question and it would not be wrong to establish people's names.

Checking for understanding

Checking for understanding would involve asking the client specific questions to ensure that the helper has a good grasp of the client's whole situation.

Focusing

Focusing can be taken to mean helping the client to explore a specific area or areas of his or her situation or problem.

Reflecting

Reflecting is a therapeutic tool which allows the client the opportunity to hear what has been said and may serve to prompt him or her to offer more information. Reflecting has also been described as a mini-summary, the basic idea however, rests with the activity of looking back and assessing the progress made by both client and helper.

Echoing

Echoing is the act of repeating the last phrase or couple of words which the client has said. Here again the purpose is to illicit further elaboration on the part of the client.

Non-verbal responding

Most non-verbal responding would accompany some form of verbal responding. These could be grouped under the term of kinesics, which was discussed in Chapter 16, and would include proxemics, gesture and posture. Touch and silence are also non-verbal ways of responding and these have already been explored in Chapter 16.

Paralanguage as a means of responding

Responding through the use of paralanguage includes such vocal utterances as 'uh', 'um', 'uh-huh', and silent pauses, all these would serve to encourage the client to talk.

Communication and helping

It could be argued that communication is a fundamental tool for health care delivery. Quality of care is in fact dictated by the effectiveness of communication which, in turn, is underpinned by self-awareness. Self-awareness as emphasised throughout this book, is the backbone of any therapeutic relationship. It is therefore a prerequisite for the professional caregiver to know and understand him or herself before venturing to embark on the helping process. The tri-dimensional nature of communication (verbal, non-verbal and paralanguage) suggests that the very act of being (that is, existing) sends out messages to others. More often than not, these messages are true reflections of one's internal dynamics. Perception of these messages dictates the nature of the interaction self has with other(s). Awareness of one's internal dynamics contributes to effective communication and in particular therapeutic communication. Three of the factors which dictate the flow and direction of interpersonal communication are listening, attending and responding. A lesson one can learn from the prisoner's dilemma (see Chapter 15) is that, 'if you risk to lose by opening your mouth, then keep it shut, at least that way, you may benefit.' In any health care setting, the focus for the helper should be on listening and attending, more so than talking.

Foundation of a therapeutic relationship

Warmth, acceptance, genuineness and empathy add a humanistic dimension to communication. W.A.G.E. is perhaps an appropriate acronym to use since it conveys the sentiment of being paid for the work that one has done. Warmth can be described as positive and affectionate feelings held **Warmth** towards another person. One could argue that to be warm is to be inviting and approachable. This in turn sows the seeds for the birth of a rapport between the helper and his or her client. Even in its literal sense, being warm conveys a positive feeling. Although it may be difficult to articulate what warm is, it can easily be perceived by others. Warmth to a patient is like honey to Pooh Bear. Despite the joviality of expression, the sentiment conveys reality.

Acceptance

Acceptance is another of those elusive concepts which Rogers (1983) used synonymously with prizing, trust and non-possessive caring, for example, accept me for who I am, not for what I can or cannot do. The three dimensions of acceptance are:

1   acceptance of self
2   acceptance of others and
3   being accepted by others

One could argue that acceptance of others rests with the acceptance of self, for example, if I cannot accept myself for who I am, it is unlikely that I can accept others for who they are. From Maslow's (1954) point of view, acceptance of self and being accepted by others can be seen as a deficiency need. The implication is that if this need is not satisfied, mental health problems will result. According to Rogers the need for acceptance is so powerful that one is prepared to sacrifice one's own organismic valuing process in the form of introjected feeling. It would be wrong to believe that everyone is accepting, in fact perhaps the reverse would be true. This implies that everyone is not accepting, until pleasing traits and characteristics are observed in others. Acceptance of self and that of others are arduous tasks that can only be achieved through intensive self-reflective skills practice underpinned by Rogers' (1951) philosophy of unconditional positive regards. Bolton (1986) highlights seven key beliefs which can facilitate the acquisition of the skills of acceptance and these are:

1   No one is perfectly accepting
2   Some tend to be more accepting than others
3   The level of acceptance in a person is constantly shifting
4   It is natural to have favourites
5   Everyone can be more accepting
6   Pseudo-acceptance is harmful to interpersonal relationships
7   Acceptance is not synonymous with approval

Genuineness

To be truly genuine means to be authentic and being able to express what one feels. This can be simply expressed as WYSIWYG 'what you see is what you get'. Bolton (1986, p.260) states, 'the genuine person knows it is impossible to be completely self-revealing, but is committed to a responsible honesty and openness with others'.

Empathy

Empathy refers to one's ability to perceive the situation from the other person's point of view. 'To sense the client's private world as if it were your own, but without ever losing the "as if" quality' (Kirschenbaum and Henderson, 1990, p.226). The ability to enter the world of another person and knowing when and where to come out is a skill which is a prerequisite in any helping relationship. Having said that, it would be dangerous to even attempt to enter the world of others if one does not have the skill and ability to enter one's own world. Self-awareness is therefore crucial to interpersonal communication. Three of the key enhancers of self-awareness are trust, disclosure and feedback, these form part of the discussion in Chapter 18.

References

Adler, R.B. and Rodman, G. (1982). *Understanding Human Communication.* London: Holt, Rinehart and Winston.

Barker, L. (1971). *Listening Behaviour.* Englewood Cliffs, NJ: Prentice-Hall.

Berne, E. (1964). *Games People Play; The Psychology of Human Relationships.* London: Penguin Books.

Bolton, R. (1986). *People Skills. 'How To Assert Yourself, Listen To Others, and Resolve Conflicts.'* Australia: Prentice-Hall.

Egan, G. (1977). *You and Me: The Skills of Communicating and Relating to Others.* Monterey, CA: Brooks/Cole.

Kirschenbaum, H. and Henderson, V.L. (1990). *The Carl Rogers Readers.* London: Constable.

McGregor, G. and White, R.S. (Eds) (1990). *Reception and Response: Hearer Creativity and the Analysis of Spoken and Written Texts.* London: Routledge.

Maslow, A.H. (1954). *Motivation and Personality.* New York: Harper.

Myers, G.E. and Myers, M.T. (1992). *The Dynamics of Human Communication: A Laboratory Approach.* London: McGraw-Hill.

Rankin, P.Y. (1926). 'Measurement of the ability to understand the spoken language.' Unpublished PhD dissertation, The University of Michigan. Cited in Myers, G.E. and Myers, M.T. (1992). *The Dynamics of Human Communication: A Laboratory Approach.* London: McGraw-Hill.

Reik, T. (1948). *Listening with the Third Ear.* New York: Arena Books.

Rogers, C.R. (1951). *Client Centred Therapy.* London: Constable.

Rogers, C.R. (1983). *Freedom to Learn for the 80's.* Columbus, OH: Charles E. Merrill.

Tedeschi, R.G. (1990). 'Therapeutic listening.' In: McGregor, G. and White, R.S. (Eds) *Reception and Response: Hearer Creativity and the Analysis of Spoken and Written Texts.* London and New York: Routledge.

Trust, disclosure, feedback and self-awareness *18*

Objectives

After reading this chapter you should be able to:

1   Explain the meaning of trust and its significance to interpersonal relationships
2   Describe some of the characteristics of trust
3   Recognise the risks involved in trusting others
4   Explain the trust–mistrust continuum
5   Describe at least one source of trust
6   Describe the various categories of disclosure
7   Explain Dinda's (1994) tri-dimensional nature of disclosure
8   Describe some of the implications of self-disclosure on mental health
9   Recognise some of the fears of self-disclosure
10 Explain how self-disclosure can be a therapeutic tool
11 Engage in your own self-disclosure
12 Explain what feedback is and is not
13 Engage in some feedback exercises
14 Describe the relationship between trust, disclosure, feedback and self-awareness

Trust

Trust can be seen as extremely important in any interpersonal relationship. We fall out with our best friends because we feel that we have been betrayed, or let down. 'I thought I knew you,' 'I never thought that you'd do this to me,' 'I thought that we were friends,' are all expressions we utter when we feel our trust has been betrayed. According to Tubbs and Moss (1994, p.180) betrayal of trust is one of the most important reasons for a low point in any intimate relationship. 'Some people are so devastated by betrayal of this kind that their loss of trust carries over into later relationships.' Trust is an abstract concept which is basically responsible for the success or failure of any person to person relationship. Tubbs and Moss define trust as the belief or feeling that no harm will come from others in a relationship. Some (Rossiter and Pearce, 1975) argue that trust can be experienced only when a relationship is characterised by:

- Contingency. If what others do affects an individual, then this individual will have a need to trust them. If this is not the case, the need to trust others will not exist.
- Predictability. Being able to predict behaviour will dictate whether or not one can trust others. For example, if my prediction leads to positive feelings then I will engage in trusting behaviour. If my prediction leads to negative feelings, I will not trust the other person. This is illustrated by Shakespeare's Julius Caesar, when referring to Cassius, Caesar remarked to Mark Antony, 'Let me have men about me that are fat, sleek-headed men, and such as sleep a nights. Yond Cassius has a lean and hungry look; He thinks too much: such men are dangerous.' Similarly if one cannot predict what others will do, trust will not be on the menu. This suggests that people have their own frame of references which they use to establish whether they should or should not trust others.
- Alternative options, here the focus is on choice. One may have other options but one chooses to trust.

Trust therefore is developed only when there is contingency, predictability and alternative options.

Whom do we trust?

Whom do we trust? This may seem a very simple question, the answer however is far from being easy. In fact one could argue that trust can only be viewed from a personal perspective. The person whom I choose to trust is not necessarily the person you will trust. Perhaps the starting point should be with self-reflection. Try Exercise 70.

Make a list of all those people you trust and note your reasons for it. Check the characteristics of those people. Compare your notes with a colleague. Make a similar list of all those people whom you do not trust and again note your reasons for it and compare notes with your colleague.

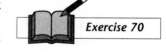

Exercise 70

Okay, you now know whom you trust, whom you do not trust and possibly some of the reasons you trust or do not trust these people. What you may find is that there are certain characteristics which are conducive to trusting behaviour. These include:

- being honest (open and sincere)
- supporting
- dependable and can be relied upon
- genuine
- warm
- accepting

The risks of trust

Trust is the foundation of all interpersonal relationship, and for this particular reason, a person may have no choice but to take the risk of opening up and sharing his or her thoughts and ideas with the others. This risk will only pay off if others reciprocate one's behaviour. The process of trust therefore involves an element of risk, because even though one perceives those qualities in others it does not necessarily follow that one's perception will be correct. People make their decision to trust or not to trust others based on how they feel and what they think of others. When I am open and vulnerable and if I am made to feel safe and protected, then I will extend the element of trust somewhat further until such time as I feel reasonably confident that I will not be hurt in the relationship. This sentiment is captured in Egan's (1977, p.172) concept of 'trust spiral'. '. . as your trust will encourage them to trust you, so their trust will enable you to trust them even further. Then, if you provide accurate understanding and receive it from others, you and the other group members will launch yourselves on the trust spiral.'

Figure 18.1

Shows the trust and mistrust continuum. After Beck, Rawlins, and Williams (1988)

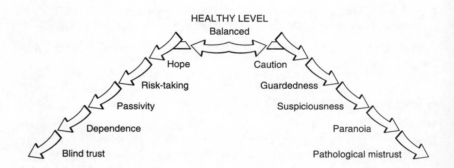

The continuum of trust and mistrust

According to Beck et al (1988) if people are to develop healthily, then their level of trust must be in equilibrium. A state of blind trust is reached when people have total reliance on others without having assessed the situation to establish whether others deserve the trust or not. Blind trust leads to total dependency and the expectation that others will always bail them out in their hour of need. The state of pathological mistrust suggests a complete lack of trust, even for those who are close to oneself. It can in fact be called a disease, and this starts from mere cautiousness and progresses to extreme paranoia (see Figure 18.1).

Learning to trust

From Erikson's theory one can deduce that trust versus mistrust is the very first conflict an infant has to resolve. The basic sentiment would suggest that if infants are able to establish an element of permanency in those who care for them, they will then feel comfortably secure. This security will further generate trust in others. This leads to the feeling that my mother does not have to be present here with me all the time, but knowing that she is always there for me, is reassuring enough. The implication of such theory leads one to conclude that trust is a learned behaviour and one does not inherit a trusting gene. The situation and the people concerned in it are appraised and conclusions are drawn as to whether they can be trusted or not. The first step of this assessment is risk taking.

Trust exercises

There are numerous trust exercises one can engage in and some of these include:

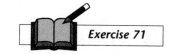
Exercise 71

- Backward fall and catch (stand few steps away and with your back to a colleague. With your eyes closed let yourself fall back and your colleague will catch you thus ensuring you do not hurt yourself. Falling backward into your colleague carries an element of risk. Having said that, if your colleague were to drop you, you would know that you cannot trust him or her to catch you).
- Forward fall and catch (this is similar to backward fall except this time you fall forward).
- Backward and forward fall and catch (this is a combination of the backward fall and forward fall and catch).
- Fall in a circle (your classmates form a tight circle, you stand in the middle with your eyes closed and you allow yourself to fall or to be gently pushed in all directions).
- Blind walk (as the name suggests you walk with your eyes closed and allow yourself to be guided by your colleague).

Disclosure and the three faces of disclosure

The word disclosure has a tendency to generate fear in people, mainly because it implies revealing information about oneself. The film *Disclosure* which stars Michael Douglas and Demi Moore, cannot have done much to allay these fears. Fortunately disclosure does not have to be taken in the context of that film. The kind of information which one can reveal falls into at least three categories. These are

- cognitive,
- affective and
- behavioural.

Cognitive information include one's thoughts, ideas, opinions, memories, past experience, and any other context within the domain of mental functioning. For example I share or disclose my thoughts with you.

Cognitive disclosure

Affective disclosure emphasises one's emotions and feelings towards either oneself or towards others, these include friends and intimate partners. For example I share or disclose my feelings with you.

Affective disclosure

Behavioural disclosure

Behavioural disclosure concerns those aspects of what one does, and, unlike the other two components, a major aspect of behavioural disclosure is self revealing. This point has been made elsewhere in the discussion of non-verbal behaviour. Behavioural disclosure can be made in either SMALL or LARGE fonts. A printing term is used here to make the point that some people are good at masking their non-verbals, whilst others can be read like a book with big print.

According to Dinda (1994) self-disclosure is a tri-dimensional concept in that it is:

1   an act
2   an interpersonal process
3   an intrapersonal process

The act of self-disclosure

Jourard (1971b) defines self-disclosure as the act of making oneself manifest so that one can be perceived by others. Whether people choose to self disclose or not is a matter for them to decide. 'If people are books, then some persons have let themselves be read from cover to cover, while others have let only the title and author's name stand forth' (Jourard, 1971b, p.2). Some find it easy to disclose, others may find it too traumatic to even think of having to disclose to another person. This act of self-disclosure is linked with personality trait. This basically means that part of one's total make up includes the willingness to disclose or not to disclose. Depending on where one is on the continuum of willingness and unwillingness to self disclose, one's personality trait could be low discloser or high discloser. Jourard believes that there is a connection between people's secretiveness and their mental health. The implication here is that the more secretive people are, the most likely they are to suffer from mental health problems. Jourard (1971a, p.6) also implied that the act of self-disclosure is a tool for self-knowledge. 'No man can come to know himself except as an outcome of disclosing himself to another person.'

The interpersonal process of self-disclosure

Self-disclosure is seen as an interpersonal process in that it forms part and parcel of an interaction between two people. Basically I meet you and as I get to know you, I start to tell you things about myself and you reciprocate. Jourard in fact believes that disclosure begets disclosure. This sounds simple but in reality is not. Reciprocity of self-disclosure is based on very important factors such as one's attitudes, values, beliefs, likes and dislikes and whether or not one trusts the other person. 'Psychotherapists have long noted that when a patient feels warmth, trust, and confidence in his therapist, he discloses himself more freely and fully than when he perceives that therapist as hostile or punitive, or when he dislikes the therapist' (Jourard, 1971b, p.13). Although reciprocity of self-disclosure does occur, nevertheless it does not occur on a tit for tat basis ('My most embarrassing moment was. . .' 'My most embarrassing moment was. .'), Dinda (1994, cited in Duck, 1994, p.33). This is like me telling you one thing about myself and you telling me a similar thing about yourself.

The intrapersonal process of self-disclosure

The intrapersonal perspective of self-disclosure is said to be grounded in its application rather than in theories or research. The argument is that self-disclosure is a gradual and incremental process which starts from a position of non-disclosure to disclosure. This is very much like starting from point 'No' and gradually working your way to point 'Yes' and in between there are the 'May be' and the 'Sometimes'. One of the deciding factors in whether one discloses or not, is trust. At the start of a relationship a person may start from a 'No' position and as the relationship develops, that person may feel more trusting of the other interactant, thus initiating the process of self-disclosure.

Self-disclosure and mental health

According to Jourard, there is a correlation between mental health state and disclosure. The implication is that disclosure is a symptom of a healthy personality and closedness is a symptom of sickness. Jourard believes that until people are true to themselves and act their real selves they will not be in a position to grow and develop. Personal growth is linked with the Jourard's concept of transparency. Jourard believed that self-disclosure is in fact necessary for personal growth. According to Littlejohn (1992) transparency has two dimensions and these are:

* allowing the world to disclose itself freely and
* the person's willingness to disclose him or herself to others

Following Jourard's publication of the concept of self-disclosure, numerous findings emerged. Littlejohn's summary of these findings include:

1   Disclosure increases with increased relational intimacy
2   Disclosure increases with reward
3   Disclosure increases the need to reduce uncertainty in a relationship
4   Disclosure tends to be reciprocal
5   Women tend to be higher disclosers than men
6   Women disclose more with individuals they like, men disclose more with people they trust

Jourard reflects that the way to a healthy mental health state is to drop one's façade and be oneself. This journey may be fraught with risk and may inspire terror, nevertheless its goal will be rewarding in that at least it enables an individual to be both mentally and physically healthy. 'Honesty can literally be a health insurance policy' (Jourard, 1971a, p,133).

The fear of self-disclosure

Why does self-disclosure generate fear or discomfort in most people? One possible reason is that the majority of people prefer to avoid talking about themselves for fear of sounding boring, or they prefer to think that they do not have anything interesting to say about themselves. They also believe that what they feel, think and do are private and would like to keep them as such. One sometimes forgets that one discloses to others all the time. Although one may not be aware of its nature or the amount of information one discloses, there is no doubt however that disclosure is ongoing. People are generally classified on a continuum of high discloser and low discloser. High disclosers tend to reveal far more about themselves than one would expect. The time and place may not necessarily be appropriate. Low disclosers on the other hand reveal as little as possible about themselves. In fact if they have the chance they would prefer not to disclose at all. Egan listed some of the reasons why people are not keen to disclose themselves more fully with others and these include:

- Family background. This is linked with learned behaviour, for example if our parents make it a habit to be open and free then we will be open and freely expressing. Similarly if our parents are closed and personal issues are not part of the daily menu then we will be inclined not to disclose ourselves to others.
- Fear of knowing oneself. As Egan (1977) said, self-disclosure can in fact put people into contact with parts of themselves that they would rather ignore.
- Fear of closeness. Deep disclosure by its very nature creates an element of closeness and it may well be that the individual does not want this closeness with the other person.
- Fear of change. Disclosure leads to awareness and awareness may mean making changes and if one does not want changes, one would prefer not to know. Not to know means not to disclose and not to disclose means one can afford to leave things as they are.
- Fear of rejection. If you get to know me as I truly am, you may not like me and if you come not to like me, you may reject me.

The appropriateness of self-disclosure

The appropriateness of self-disclosure is based on the following factors:

- How much to disclose?
- How deep to disclose?
- How much time to spend on self-disclosure?
- Whom to disclose to?
- Where to disclose, what situation and in what context?

To put it crudely, self-disclosure is inappropriate when instead of dumping his or her baggage onto you, the client leaves, taking with him or her your baggage as well. In this instance self-disclosure becomes non-therapeutic.

Self-disclosure as a therapeutic tool

Disclosure can be used as a tool for helping clients to disclose. The helper's self-disclosure can help to clarify the client's own feelings and thoughts. 'An intuitive, introverted type of patient sadly remembers difficulty with differentiating right from left, along with physical discomfort in the real world and incomprehension when required to learn kinaesthetically. The psychotherapist bends down to show the scar on her leg which she used as a little girl to help her decide which side was left. This moment is unforgettable; the bonding, person to person. Yet it is enacted by a professional person who, at that very moment, has taken responsibility for that self-disclosure in the psychotherapy, judging it appropriate and timely to trust or delight the patient with a sense of shared personhood. The two then become siblings in comprehension, siblings in discovery, and siblings in the quest for wholeness' (Clarkson and Pokorny, 1994, p.338). One can deduce from this that self-disclosure does not have to be deep to be helpful. Any personal information which can enhance the helping relationship should be offered to the client, provided the helper is comfortable with it. The major issue is the appropriateness of the helper's self-disclosure and any situation which leads to 'I come to you with one problem and leave with two problems, yours plus mine' should be avoided. There is within most clients an element of needing to know certain things about the helper. So long as self-disclosure is appropriate, it will enhance the authenticity of the relationship between the client and helper.

Jourard (1971a, p.134), argues that clients are most likely to accept the invitation to self disclose when the therapist shows uncontrived honesty. However when the therapist is authentically a person who means well, he or she will come across as such and 'the need for sneaky projective tests or for decoding hidden messages in utterances vanishes, the patient then wants to make himself known, and proceeds to do so. In this defenceless state, the interpretations, suggestions, and advice of the therapist then have maximum, growth-yielding impact on him.'

Skills practice of self-disclosure

Although the sentiments that have been reflected thus far seem to suggest an element of hereditary, that is a personality trait, nevertheless one can argue that the ability to disclose is also a skill. And as with all skills, in order to get better the professional caregiver needs to practice. There are numerous ways of improving ones self-disclosure skills, some of these will be highlighted here. All these exercises are meant to involve the reader and at least one other person, the preparation for self-disclosure however can be done on an individual basis.

- Make a list of at least 20 sentences, each starting with 'I am . . .' (I know that sometimes this can be difficult especially if you seldom self reflect. Having said that, one needs to bear in mind that self-disclosure is one's insurance policy for a healthy state of being).

Egan's 'I am' exercise

Exercise 72

- Review your list and decide which of those statements you think are appropriate to disclose. Explore your rationale for those statements which you feel are inappropriate, such as for whom are they inappropriate, you or your colleagues or the group? Think about the timing, the situation, how long you have known the other person and so on.
- Engage (in turn you and your colleague or group members) in disclosing those appropriate self-statements.

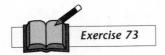

Exercise 73

Work through the stages of the experiential learning process and enrich the knowledge of your 'self'.

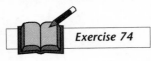

I'll tell you one thing about me and you tell me one thing about you

Exercise 74

The 'I'll tell you one thing about me and you tell me one thing about you,' is as simple as it sounds. There are no hidden agendas or tricks, just select one person from your group and engage in the exercise. For example I could start with, 'My name is . . . ,' You then respond with one of your own answers. Let the process continue until you feel you have exhausted what you feel is appropriate to disclose. Again as with all those exercises, it is much more beneficial to process it through the concept of experiential learning.

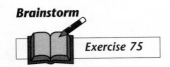

Brainstorm

Exercise 75

As a group, brainstorm some ideas as to what sort of things you could disclose. Make a note of these and ask each member to select one or two statements he or she feels comfortable to disclose. Complete the process through the stages of experiential learning.

Each member should choose any three items, which reveal his or her:

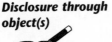
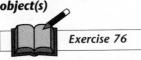

Disclosure through object(s)

Exercise 76

- Philosophy, culture, and such like
- Taste, for instance in music, food and any other area
- Relationships

In turn tell your colleagues about yourself through these items.

The above are intended as guides to what sort of things you can choose to explore. As a group you can be as creative as you feel, as long as everyone feels comfortable with what they have to engage in. Review this exercise through the stages of experiential learning process.

Feedback

From a simplistic perspective, feedback can be seen as a response to a listener. As Myers and Myers (1992) say, feedback is an integral part of any transaction and can be represented in both one's verbal and non-verbal cues. Egan (1977) sees feedback as being told by others what you are doing right, so that you can continue to do it, and what you are doing wrong, so that you can stop it. One could argue that feedback is a basic need, which is not too dissimilar to Maslow's concept of cognitive need. Here however the focus is on the need to know what others think of oneself. Feedback therefore is a prerequisite for any person to person relationships and it serves as an important source of information about oneself. Used properly, feedback is the mirror which reflects one's thoughts, feelings and actions, and this can actually enhance both one's physical and psychological well-being.

- Feedback is about behaviour (like giving me information about my teaching)
- Feedback is not about the person (not about me as the person)
- Feedback seeks to change a behaviour (my teaching style)
- Feedback does not seek to change the person (not me)
- Feedback is meant to enhance growth and development (enhance my self-concept)
- Feedback is not meant to be a put-down (destructive criticism)
- Feedback is given only when asked for (tell me what do you think of my approach to this subject)
- Feedback is not forced (I will tell you what I think of you whether you ask for it or not)
- Feedback is about observations (say what you see)
- Feedback is not about inferences (do not say what you feel or think)
- Feedback is descriptive
- Feedback is not evaluative
- Feedback is given sensitively, honestly and with a sentiment of genuine concern for the other person
- Feedback is specific, not woolly or fuzzy
- Feedback is immediate, not delayed
- Feedback is given about aspects of behaviour that can be changed
- Feedback is personalised (as in I, me and my and not the group, we, etc.)

Dynamics between trust, disclosure, feedback and self-awareness

The dynamic between trust, disclosure and feedback is demonstrated in Luft's (1969) concept of Johari Window (discussed in Chapter 2). A very brief reflection on Johari Window leads to the following conclusion about the way one's experiences are structured. An individual can be viewed as consisting of four quadrants and these are:

1 open self (known to self and known to others)
2 blind self (unknown to self and known to others)
3 hidden self (known to self and unknown to others)
4 unknown self (unknown to self and unknown to others)

Self-awareness is the key issue in determining the size of these quadrants. If for example I am limited in self-awareness, then it is most likely that the size of my four quadrants will look something like Figure 18.2, where my open self is clouded by my blind self.

Imagine the following scenario: 'I have developed a very good relationship with you and your behaviour (verbal and non-verbal) leads me to conclude that I can really trust you. Because of this trust, I find myself able to disclose more freely to you. My disclosure will lead you to get to know me better than before. Here you have the advantage of being more objective about me than I would be about myself. When I ask you for feedback on my behaviour, theoretically you will be better placed to give it. Some of the feedback you give will be known and some unknown to me.'

Here is another one of those 'it really happened to me' stories. One day I asked one of my groups of students to give me some feedback about my behaviour as a lecturer and I was pleasantly surprised to hear that I had a tendency to gaze more to my left than to my right. Reflecting on my behaviour I concluded that my students were right. I started from the blind perspective (i.e.) unknown to self and known to others, and through feedback from my students I was able to progress to the open perspective (i.e.) known to self and others.

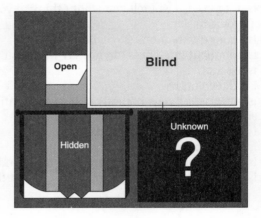

Figure 18.2
Johari Window showing lack of self-awareness

This is just one piece of information which has shifted from my blind self to my open self, thus reducing the size of my blind quadrant and enlarging my open quadrant. Whenever there is this type of dynamics between trust disclosure and feedback within interpersonal relationships, one's open self gradually increases, leaving the other three quadrants to become smaller and smaller (see Figure 18.3).

The point has been made before that self-awareness has no boundary and as such is a never-ending process. This would mean that an individual's open quadrant can never truly become one whole quadrant thus replacing the three other quadrants. There will always be a blind, hidden and an unknown quadrant in one's existence. One's goal, through self-awareness, is to continually increase one's open self.

Feedback exercises

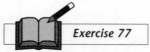

Exercise 77

Reflect on any one or two situations in your life when you were given feedback and make notes of the following points:

- Who was it from?
- How was it given (what was actually said?)
- How did you feel after?
- How did you respond?

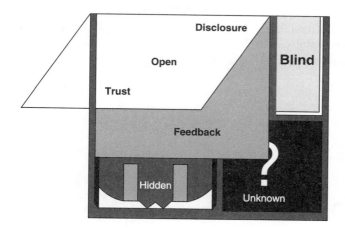

Figure 18.3
Shows the effect of self-awareness on an individual's Johari Window. Note the size of the open quadrant

This exercise could serve as a guide as to how feedback should be, if for example you felt uncomfortable with the feedback you received, then obviously there would be a big question mark over the effectiveness of the feedback. On the other hand if you feel good about what was said, this could be indicative of how effective the feedback was. The issue of receiving feedback in the form of criticism is dealt with in Chapter 19.

References

Beck, C.K., Rawlins, R.P. and Williams, S.R. (1988). *Mental Health Psychiatric Nursing: A Holistic Life-cycle Approach*. St. Louis, MO: Mosby.

Clarkson, P. and Pokorny, M. (Eds) (1994). *The Handbook of Psychotherapy*. London and New York: Routledge and Kegan Paul.

Dinda, K. (1994). 'The intrapersonal interpersonal dialectical process of self-disclosure.' In: Duck, S. (Ed.) *Dynamics of Relationships*. Thousand Oaks, London, New Delhi: Sage.

Duck, S. (Ed.) (1994). *Dynamics of Relationships*. Thousand Oaks, London, New Delhi: Sage.

Egan, G. (1977). *You and Me: The Skills of Communicating and Relating to Others*. Monterey CA: Brooks/Cole.

Erikson, H. (1963). *Childhood and Society*. New York: Norton.

Jourard, S.M. (1971a). *The Transparent Self*. New York: Van Nostrand Reinhold.

Jourard, S.M. (1971b). *Self-Disclosure: An Experimental Analysis of the Transparent Self*. New York: Wiley-Interscience.

Littlejohn, S. (1992). *The Theories of Human Communication*. Belmont, CA: Wadsworth.

Luft, J. (1969). *Of Human Interaction*. Palo Alto, CA: National Press.

Myers, G.E. and Myers, M.T. (1992). *The Dynamics of Human Communication: A Laboratory Approach*. London: McGraw-Hill.

Rossiter, C.M. and Pearce, W.B. (1975). *Communicating Personally*. Indianapolis, IN: Bobbs-Merrill.

Tubbs, S.L. and Moss, S. (1994). *Human Communication*. London: McGraw-Hill.

Assertiveness and caring 19

Objectives

After reading this chapter you should be able to:

1. Define the term assertiveness
2. Differentiate between assertiveness, submissiveness, and aggressiveness
3. List some of the basic human rights
4. Explain some of the benefits of being:
   a. assertive
   b. submissive and
   c. aggressive
5. Explain some of the types of assertion
6. Engage in some assertive skills practice
7. List and explain some of the do's and dont's of assertive response
8. Give and receive criticisms
9. Describe some of the implications for care delivery

Definition of terms

There is a common misconception about assertive behaviour. Those who behave assertively are often perceived as aggressive and those who behave aggressively perceive themselves as assertive. Some irrational thinking such as, 'to be aggressive is to be assertive', or 'being assertive is uncaring' are still apparent in the way people behave. In many ways, perhaps it is not that difficult to see why there is so much ambiguity about the concept of assertiveness, since theorists and writers on the subject have their own particular definition of what assertive behaviour is about. As Rakos (1991, p.7) points out, 'a striking demonstration of the lack of conceptual clarity characterising assertiveness is provided by St. Lawrence (1987), who identified more than 20 distinctly different definitions presently used in research and training'. Strangely however, none of the definitions point to either being aggressive or being uncaring. Some of the definitions of assertiveness include:

- 'Behaviour which enables a person to act in his own best interests, to stand up for himself without undue anxiety, to express his honest feelings comfortably, or to exercise his own rights without denying the rights of others we call *assertive behaviour*' (Alberti and Emmons, 1970, p.2).

- 'Being assertive means actually putting the skills you have into practice. An assertive person steers a middle course between not doing anything and doing too much. An assertive person gets the work of interpersonal communication done but does so in a way that respects both his or her own rights and the rights of others' (Egan, 1977, p.39).
- 'Standing up for your own rights in such a way that you do not violate another person's rights. Expressing your needs, wants, opinions, feelings and beliefs in direct, honest and appropriate ways' (Back and Back, 1991, p.1).

Assertiveness

The basic sentiment of these definitions seems to suggest that being assertive means safeguarding one's rights in such a way as not to infringe the rights of others and being able to express oneself clearly, confidently and honestly. One could say that an assertive person would adopt the 'I'm OK – you're OK life position,' 'I win and you win'. One of the main distinctions between assertiveness and submissiveness is that in the case of the latter, one demonstrates a lack of confidence in one's behaviour and this results in one's rights being violated. A classic example of such behaviour would be the inability to say no to a request or feeling guilty after having said no to such a request. As Back and Back (1991, p.2) succinctly put it, 'expressing your needs, wants, opinions, feelings, and beliefs in apologetic, diffident, or self-effacing ways'. I let you have your own way even if I am inconvenienced in the process. The life positions would be, 'I'm not OK and you're OK,' 'I lose and you win'. Some examples of such behaviour include:

Submissiveness

- Saying 'I'm sorry' even if it is not your fault
- Accepting the blame even if you are not responsible
- Always behaving in a way which gives the impression that others are superior to yourself
- The word 'no' does not exist in your vocabulary

Alberti and Emmons (1970) state that the non-assertive person is likely to think of the appropriate response after the opportunity has passed.

Aggressiveness

The main differentiation between aggressiveness and assertiveness is that in the case of the former, the behaviour suggests a lack of respect for others. Here the emphasis is on satisfying one's own needs at the expense of others and obviously violating their rights in the process. I stand for my rights and that is all I concern myself with. The scenario here is, 'I'm OK and you're not OK,' 'I win and you lose'.

Some examples of such behaviour include:

- Being verbally abusive
- Being physically abusive
- Behaving in a manner which conveys an element of superiority towards others
- Being sarcastic (this could be seen as indirect aggression)

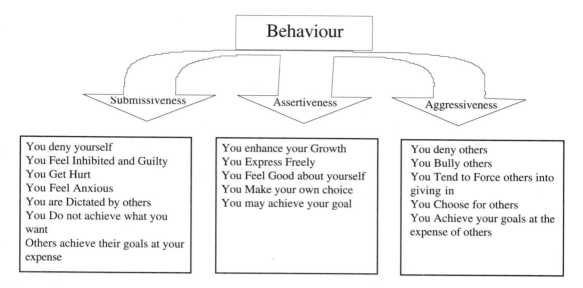

Figure 19.1

The contrast of feelings elicited by submissive, assertive and aggressive behaviours can be seen in Figure 19.1.

A contrast of behaviours between Submissiveness, Assertiveness and Aggressiveness

A question of rights

At the very heart of assertiveness lies the issue of 'rights'. It goes without saying therefore that if people do not know what their rights are then it is unlikely that they will know what or how to protect these. What are these rights then? A dictionary definition of the word 'right' suggests, 'just, required by morality or equity or duty' (*The Pocket Oxford Dictionary of Current English*, 1984, p.643). The implication here is that this 'thing' is owed to us, it belongs to us and it is morally ours. This being the case, what are these 'things' which are morally ours? Before exploring these rights, try Exercise 78.

Make a list of all those things which you consider you are morally entitled to.

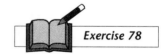

Exercise 78

Some basic human rights

There are numerous rights which you may have come up with, the main ones however are focused around the concept of basic human rights and these include:

*   The right to say no if that is what you want (like refusing a request)
*   The right to be you
*   The right to change your mind
*   The right to respect
*   The right to make your own choices

- The right to express your opinions and your beliefs
- The right to do anything you want as long as it does not interfere with the rights of others
- The right to make the occasional mistake
- The right to express your needs and desires
- The right to choose whether you want to be assertive or not
- The right to remain silent
- The right to information
- The right to have control over your body
- The right to have control over your possessions
- The right to make your own decisions
- The right to education
- The right to fair treatment
- The right to say 'I don't understand'
- The right to question
- The right to decline responsibility which you are not prepared to take

Some benefits of submissiveness

There is a belief, although absurd as it may sound, that some people find certain benefits in allowing their rights to be violated. Some of these benefits include:

- Avoiding conflict, like being left in peace and quiet
- Being approved by others
- Being accepted because you come across as nice and dependable

Some benefits of aggressiveness

The benefits of being aggressive are easier to conceptualise and some of these include:

- Venting feelings of anger
- Fewer chances of your rights being violated
- More often you get what you want
- Feeling of domination
- Feeling superior to others
- Ignoring or dismissing the behaviour of others

Some benefits of assertiveness

There is little doubt that the benefits of being assertive far outweigh those of aggressiveness and submissiveness. Some of these benefits include:

- Being respected for being honest and fair
- Developing a sense of self-respect
- Having a personal sense of value and positive self-esteem
- Having the ability to establish good interpersonal relationships with others
- Being able to satisfy your own needs
- Not having to have to think of excuses to justify your reasons for having said no
- Never having to be in the role of the victim

- Being in charge of your own feelings
- Feeling a sense of independence

Types of assertion

There are numerous types of assertion and some of these include:

- Direct or basic assertion, which involves actually making one's position clear in a direct and straightforward manner.
- Indirect assertion is focused around not actually 'saying no' but the 'no' sentiment is left for others to pick up, for example I would tell you that I have a lot on, I have to do this, that and the other, but I do not come out and actually tell you 'no I won't go out for a drink'.
- Empathic assertion suggests that the assertive person demonstrates the ability to understand any situation from the other person's point of view, while at the same time making it clear that certain things will have to be done. For example, as my boss, you want me to complete a workload analysis questionnaire, which I have difficulty with, due to lack of time. I put my case forward and having listened to me, you respond with the following statement. 'I do understand how you must feel, having to complete the workload analysis on top of everything else that you have to do, however, there is very little we can do until the policy is changed.'
- Discrepancy assertion, which according to Back and Back (1991, p.60) is 'pointing out the discrepancy between what has previously been agreed and what is actually happening or about to happen'. An example can be illustrated in the following statement. 'We have discussed in our ground rules that we would respect the opinions of each and every member of this group, what I am finding now is that this is not happening. I would like to establish exactly what our situation is.'
- Praise assertion means basically complimenting the other person for their request but at the same time refusing to engage. An example would be, 'it is very good of you to think of me, unfortunately I have to decline the offer'.
- Compromise assertion suggests that I cannot help you but I know someone who can.

From these different types of assertion, one could conclude that being assertive does not necessarily mean saying a categorical 'no'. What it does mean however is that you do what you feel is right so long as you are not inconvenienced and the other person's rights are not interfered with. There are certain situations where it may be appropriate to say 'no' to a request but that does not mean that seeking an alternative solution is out of the question. Similarly there is no problem with the use of the phrase 'I'm sorry' before turning down a request, the problem however is when 'I'm sorry' is used in abundance.

Assertive skills practice

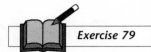

Exercise 79

Reflect on yourself and make a list of all your positive attributes.

There will be a certain element of hesitation in highlighting those positive attributes simply because you may feel this is too contrived. Having said that it would be fair to believe that being assertive is about being self confident. The starting point of any discussion on the subject of assertion rests with one's self-concept. It can be further hypothesised that there is a positive correlation between self-concept and assertive behaviour. This means that if one has a good self-concept, for example positive perception of body image, positive self-esteem and a congruence between ideal self and true self, it is most likely that one will adopt assertive behaviour. It follows that if one feels confident in oneself, the chances are that one will behave confidently. Similarly if one does not feel confident, one will not behave in a confident manner. Assertiveness is about having confidence in one's conviction, therefore to be assertive is to believe in oneself.

Do's and don'ts of assertiveness

- Do not allow your behaviour to be influenced by a 'Be perfect' driver (see Chapter 3) as this will lead you to seek an unachievable goal. Restructure your thinking to use the counter-driver of 'be yourself,' this way there is less chance of feeling inferior.
- Do not allow your behaviour to be influenced by a 'please others' driver as this will lead you to feel inferior if others are displeased with you. Use the counter-driver of 'Be selfish sometimes,' you will come to realise that you are as important as the next person. This being the case, you will learn to respect yourself and your needs more.
- Take responsibility for what you say by using 'I' statements.
- Take responsibility for the way you feel and let others be in charge of their feelings. If you feel guilty or sad, you cannot hold others responsible for these feelings. These are your feelings and you are responsible for them. For example, no one makes me feel the way I do, therefore I should not blame others.
- If you need to confront others, then do so with factual information.
- Let there be congruence between your verbals and non-verbals. Say what you mean and mean what you say. Let your body posture, gestures and facial expression tell the same story that you have in mind.
- Assertion may not always be appropriate, in which case you have to decide how you would deal with the situation. Whatever you decide, avoid escalation of conflict which may lead to bad consequences, a classic example is 'road rage'. A simple philosophy is that if it is a choice between life (adopting a submissive stance) and death (standing for one's rights no matter what), I would choose the former because I see life as more important than violation of one of

my rights. Others may feel differently and that would be quite in order.

- Display the 'broken record' behaviour. Here all you have to do is to repeat what you have said before if the other person persists with his or her request, as for example:
  No, I don't want my drive paved
  No, I am not interested
  I am not changing my mind on what I've already said.
  Let your needle be stuck in the same groove for however long it takes to get the message across, it does work, because at the end of the day no one wants to be faced with a person who has already made up his or her mind.
- Maintain eye contact when you are speaking with the other person.
- Use the correct paralanguage.

Receiving criticism

In dealing with criticism, one of the most important things is to listen to what is being said. Analyse what is being said and check if there is some truth in it, if there is, then acknowledge this. Say for example your personal tutor were to justifiably criticise your lateness, in which case acknowledge, accept and apologise for this. If however there is no truth in what the other person has said, then take it that it is the other person's perception of the events and point out that this is his or her perspective on the situation and whilst you respect his or her point of view, you do not agree with it. If negative feedback is given, and you feel you do not deserve it, then let your thinking process be like a filter, through which all the negative things can be recognised as 'not fitting' and disposed of. If it does not belong to you, then do not take it on board. These sentiments can be summarised as follows.

- Listen to what is being said
- Acknowledge what is being said
- Reflect on what has been said
- Analyse what you have heard
- Decide if it fits and
- Accept or
- Reject the feedback

Assertiveness and health care delivery

The demand for an assertive workforce is perhaps greater in health care professions than in any other professional arena. The concept of caring suggests that the helper or carer has to safeguard the health and welfare of the client. The simple rationale for the need of an assertive team to occupy this role is that being a patient one may not necessarily know or recognise what one's rights are. The helper therefore has to ensure that the

**Helper as the advocate
to the client**

**Helper as the source of
inspiration**

patient is aware of those rights. If the helper does not possess assertive attributes, then it is unlikely that he or she will be able to safeguard the health and welfare of the patient. Say for example I cannot stand up for my rights then how would I be able to stand up for someone else's rights. If I cannot look after myself, would I be able to look after you? This is very unlikely and as such it is difficult to imagine how a non-assertive person could fulfil the role of patients' advocate.

An unassertive helper is not going to instil confidence in the clients, in fact the reverse would probably take place. An aggressive helper will generate fear in the client to the point that this will be detrimental to the client's growth and development. A submissive helper casts doubt in the minds of clients regarding his or her efficiency. If you are faced with a lecturer who comes across as submissive, would you have confidence in that person's ability to do his or her job? You will most likely not have confidence in your lecturer and a similar principle would apply in the helper–client interaction. An aggressive helper would be classed as either degenerate or perverted (see Chapter 20) depending on what his or her intention is. Whichever label one uses, the fact remains that this particular practitioner will be non-therapeutic in his or her approach to care. The concepts of therapeutic and non-therapeutic are explored in Chapter 20.

References

Alberti, R.E. and Emmons, M.L. (1970). *Your Perfect Right: A Guide to Assertive Behaviour*. San Luis Obispo, CA: Impact.

Back, K. and Back, K. (1991). *Assertiveness at Work*. London: McGraw-Hill.

Egan, G. (1977). *You and Me: The Skills of Communicating and Relating to Others*. Monterey CA: Brooks/Cole.

The Pocket Oxford Dictionary of Current English (1984). 7th edn. Edited by R.E. Allen. Oxford: Clarendon Press.

Rakos, R.F. (1991). *Communication: Assertive Behaviour, Theory, Research, and Training*. London: Routledge and Kegan Paul.

Heron's six-category intervention analysis

20

Objectives

After reading this chapter you should be able to:

1 Define Heron's notion of an intervention
2 Differentiate between therapeutic and non-therapeutic intervention
3 List and explain all the non-therapeutic interventions
4 Describe some of the assessment criteria for a valid therapeutic intervention
5 Differentiate between authoritative and facilitative interventions
6 Describe all six types of interventions

The concept of intervention

To intervene is to 'interfere, modify course or result of events; come in as extraneous thing; be situated between others' (*The Pocket Oxford Dictionary of Current English*, 1984, p.386). One therefore intervenes in an attempt to change or redirect a course of action. In the context of health care delivery, intervention would mean the act of redirecting the client or patient's path, so that he or she can live as independent a life as possible. From Heron's (1990, p.3) perspective, an intervention is 'an identifiable piece of verbal and/or non-verbal behaviour that is part of the practitioner's service to the client'. Heron sees a practitioner as anyone who offers a professional service to a client. This would include such disciplines as nurses, doctors, dentists, psychiatrists, psychologists, counsellors and so on. A client on the other hand is seen as the person who is 'freely choosing (in most cases) to avail him or herself of the practitioner's service, in order to meet some need which he or she has identified' (Heron, 1990, p.1).

Practitioner

Client

Any intervention which carries the sentiment of enhancing growth and development on the part of the client is considered as a therapeutic activity. The sole objective of a therapeutic intervention is to see the client benefiting from the service which is offered. Having said that, it would be unrealistic to believe that every practitioner has the client's interest at heart. Beverly Allit would be a case in point to support my lack of faith in the human race. Any intervention which inhibits the client's growth and development is classed as non-therapeutic.

Intervention as a therapeutic activity

Consider the following 10 interventions and place a tick as you see appropriate for each, in the therapeutic or non-therapeutic column.

No.	Interventions	Therapeutic	Non-therapeutic
1	There is always a light at the end of the tunnel		
2	How are you feeling now?		
3	Look on the bright side, things couldn't get any worse		
4	I think you should be stronger and don't let it get to you		
5	Don't worry, it will soon be over		
6	Would you like me to sit with you?		
7	You shouldn't blame yourself		
8	Would you like to talk about it?		
9	It's no good looking back now, what's done is done		
10	We are doing the best we can		

Close analysis reveals that statements 1, 3, 4, 5, 7, 9 and 10 are all non-therapeutic interventions. The rationales are as follows.

'There is always a light at the end of the tunnel' suggests that everything will be okay. This would be a wrong message to give the patient because there is no guarantee that things will in fact be okay.

'Look on the bright side, things couldn't get any worse' indicates that things are really bad especially if this is being validated by the helper, who is the authority in that field.

'I think you should be stronger and don't let it get to you' implies that the patient is being weak and passive in allowing 'it to get to him or her'.

'Don't worry, it will soon be over,' sounds as if the act of worrying is conscious and under voluntary control.

'You shouldn't blame yourself' focuses on where the blame should be rather than acknowledging how the patient feels.

'It's no good looking back now, what's done is done' implies that one should forget about the past.

'We are doing the best we can,' suggests that we cannot do anymore than what we are already doing. This may mean that we are not in control of the situation.

Heron classifies non-therapeutic interventions into two main categories and these are:

- degenerate and
- perverted.

Degenerate interventions

Degenerate interventions are those interventions which occur as a result of the practitioner's incompetence. Heron (1990, p.9) in fact defines it as, 'one that fails in one, and usually several, of these respects, because the practitioner lacks personal development, or training, or experience, or awareness, or some combination of these.' This, however, does not mean that the practitioner intends to cause harm to the client. Instead the former may be out of touch with current practices and hence is apt to make mistakes. According to Heron, the source of degenerate interventions rests in lack of awareness and lack of experience. There are at least four kinds of degenerate interventions and these are:

1   Unsolicited
2   Manipulative
3   Compulsive
4   Unskilled

Unsolicited intervention suggests that the practitioner appoints him or herself to the role of helper and starts to function in that role. In a health care scenario, this would be like giving clients or patients advice which they have not asked for. A bogus doctor or a bogus paramedic may fit that description.

Unsolicited intervention

Manipulative intervention is the situation where the practitioner's focus is very much on what he or she wants rather than what the client wants. Heron (1990, p.145) says that classic examples are shown in situations where the practitioner manipulates the client 'to get sex, money or the satisfaction of power play'. In a counselling situation a manipulative intervention would be when the counsellor steers the client to talk about things which are of special interest to him or her, like details of the client's sexual life.

Manipulative interventions

Compulsive intervention occurs where the practitioner has unsolved and unacknowledged problems of his or her own. Some of the traits of compulsive helpers are:

Compulsive interventions

•   They are limited in what they can do
•   They work too hard
•   They offer help to too many people
•   They take on an unrealistic level of responsibility
•   They suffer bouts of guilt

Compulsive helpers offer three basic kinds of intervention, there are:

•   Aggressive (as in punishing, attacking and abusing the clients)
•   Pampering (as in treating the client as they are invalid)
•   Ignoring (as in avoiding or overlooking the client)

Unskilled, which basically means an incompetent practitioner due to lack of training skills.

Unskilled intervention

Reflect on your clinical or personal experiences and see if you can recognise some of the degenerate interventions which some practitioners may have been involved in. The whole purpose of this exercise is to raise your

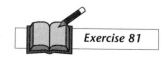

Exercise 81

awareness in terms of recognising these interventions. You may wish to discuss with your colleagues what action you may take if you encounter such interventions.

Perverted interventions

Perverted interventions are those interventions which deliberately seek to cause harm to the clients. Manipulative intervention which although falls in the category of degenerate, can have elements of perverted interventions. These are purposeful in intent and malicious in nature. This is basically, a wicked practitioner, whose objective is to seek self-satisfaction to the detriment of the clients. Although it may seem an over-generalisation, nevertheless, one could say that all those who are found guilty of professional misconduct would fit in this category.

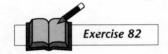
Exercise 82

Again reflect on your clinical practice or personal experience and see if you can recognise such interventions. Discuss these with a colleague and you may wish to decide on a course of action if you are faced with such an intervention.

Valid and invalid interventions

By their very nature both these interventions (i.e. degenerate and perverted) would be seen as invalid because they do not fit into the criteria for a valid intervention. Heron (1990, p.9) defines a valid intervention as one which is 'appropriate to the client's current state of development, and to the developing practitioner–client interaction'.

The criteria for a valid intervention can be highlighted as follows.

- It should be the right intervention within the right category
- Delivery should be in context and appropriate to the needs of the client
- Timing should be good

Assessment criteria for a valid therapeutic intervention

From a practical point of view, certain key questions could form part of a set of criteria for any valid therapeutic intervention. These are:

1 Awareness of the client and awareness of self
  Am I aware of the client?
  Am I listening, hearing, seeing and sensing the client?
  Am I aware of the client's whole being (i.e.) physical self, affective self, cognitive self, social self, philosophical self and any other aspects of the client's self including sexual self?
2 What cues am I picking up?

Are my values, beliefs and attitudes influencing my judgements?
Am I ware of the effect the client is having on me?
3   What do I expect from the client?
Is my expectation congruent with the client's needs?
4   Am I honest and genuine?
Do I have the client's interests at heart?
Or am I satisfying my own needs?
Are my intentions honest and sincere or am I being perverted?
5   Am I empowering or disempowering my client?
Am I leading my client to a state of helplessness?

These are just a few of the questions which , as a practitioner one can ask oneself to ensure that the interventions are growth enhancing on the part of the clients.

Six-category interventions

Heron acknowledges Blake and Mouton (1972) for their inspiration of his concept of six-category analysis of counselling interventions. As the name suggests, Heron identified six categories of interventions and these are grouped under two main classes which are:

* authoritative and
* facilitative.

Authoritative interventions

The word authority suggests an element of knowledge and influence which is attributed to someone. Authoritative does not mean wielding the rod of power to beat the client into submission. It has a much gentler meaning in the context of practitioner–client interaction. In this respect, the practitioner is the one with the authority and his or her primary role is to use that knowledge and expertise to enhance the client's therapeutic growth and development. The focus of the intervention is on the practitioner as the leader in this partnership. This however does not mean that the client has more of a passive role, on the contrary, he or she remains active through his or her care. Three categories of interventions which are underpinned by an authoritative mode of helping are:

1   Prescriptive intervention, which seeks to direct the client's behaviour
2   Informative intervention, which seeks to impart information to the client
3   Confronting intervention, which seeks to raise the client's awareness regarding his or her blind spots

Facilitative interventions

To facilitate is to make easy, the role of the practitioner therefore is to help the client through his or her situation. The focus is on the client, who has the leading role in directing his or her care, the practitioner however provides help and support. There are three categories of intervention which are grouped in facilitative mode. These are:

4   Cathartic intervention, which seeks to vent painful emotions
5   Catalytic intervention, which seeks to encourage the client into self-discovery and problem solving behaviours
6   Supportive intervention, which seeks to affirm the client's worth

Prescriptive interventions

Those from the non-directive school of thought would perhaps not agree with the concept of prescriptive intervention. These are times however, when asking the client to think or act in a certain way may be of tremendous value to that person.

> Radiographers would have to ask clients to stand or lie in a certain way so that they can be X-rayed
> Nurses would have to ask patients not to eat for a certain length of time prior to surgery
> Dentists would have to ask patients to open their mouths so that their teeth can be cleaned
> Doctors would have to ask patients to breath in and out so that they can be examined
> Physiotherapists would have to ask patients to perform some sort of activities to evaluate their progress

Although these are simplistic examples, the sentiments they convey, cannot be ignored. Having said that, the manner in which prescriptive interventions are given can make all the difference to whether they are therapeutic or non-therapeutic. There are in fact numerous ways of asking someone to do something. Try Exercise 83.

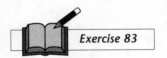
Exercise 83

Reflect on your clinical or personal experience and make a list of all verbal or non-verbal behaviour which could be classed as prescriptive interventions. I will start you off with the following.

Every time you feel anxious, I would like you to make a note of the following:

What could the possible causes be?
Your feelings and thoughts during that time
How long does the episode last?
What do you do during that time?
What makes it better?

Prescriptive interventions are seen as a behavioural approach to caring and you may have gathered from your examples that there is more than one way of 'asking'. Heron highlights the following words and phrases as prescriptive interventions.

1   Advise, for example, I would advise you take a fortnight's break from your work
2   Propose. What I propose is that you think about it over the weekend and let me know what you decide to do
3   Recommend. I recommend that you have a low fat diet
4   Suggest. I suggest you discuss this with your partner
5   Request certain behaviour from the client. I request that you refrain from smoking as of now
6   Instruct. My instructions are to be followed in order to avoid further complications
7   Demand. I demand that you stop behaving indecently otherwise you will be discharged from our care
8   Order. I order you to leave now but you may come back tomorrow
9   Command. I command you to stay in hospital under the Mental Health Act of 1983.

The latter four (i.e.) instruct, demand, order and command are seen as extreme ways of prescribing, nevertheless these are legitimate. It could be said that if other words or phrases can be used instead of instruct, demand, order and command, then these would be much more appropriate, because from a client's perspective, it does not matter how diplomatic or tactful the practitioner is, if these words are used, there is a risk of souring the relationship. This can be counter-productive and would question the therapeutic value of such interventions.

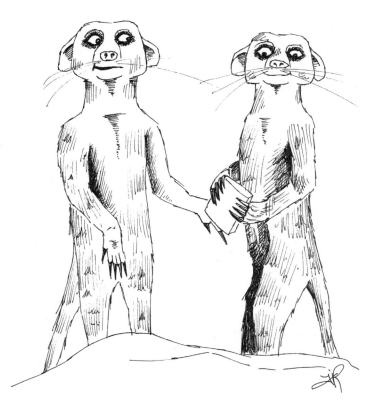

'Here is a copy of Interpersonal Communication and Psychology for Health Care Professionals, *I recommend chapter 20'*

Informative interventions

Any activity which offers new knowledge or insight to the client can be classed as informative. Clients would perceive this information as necessary to their needs and interests. Heron focuses on the following ways of offering informative interventions:

- Practitioner's rationale. Here practitioners offer a rationale for what they are doing to the clients. This, Heron (1990, p.38) says, extends from giving 'medicine through to psychotherapy and education to any professional role'.

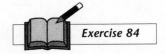

Exercise 84

Reflect on your clinical practice and make a list of all the situations which involve offering some sort of rationale to clients. One such situation could be when a nurse explains to the client why the latter is prescribed bed rest.

- Physical diagnosis and prognosis. Here the practitioner gives the client information regarding what he has discovered and what the likely outcome is going to be.
- Personal interpretation. This could involve giving some meaning to the client' behaviour, experience or situation. The main argument here is should the practitioner interpret the patient's behaviour, or would it be better for the patient to come up with his own interpretation. Again this is dependent on the practitioner's philosophical stance and method of working. What is clear however is that there should be a balanced interpretation of the client's situation, as Heron (1990) says, if you give too much explanation, no matter how accurate it is, the patient becomes a cognitive puppet. Similarly if you give too little explanation, 'the client may improperly wallow in nescience'.
- Psychosocial prediction. Here the practitioner offers possible explanations as to what may happen in certain situations. Prediction can of course be applied to situations other than the psychosocial domain, for example, 'reducing your body weight will help you breathe easier'.
- Educational and growth assessment. The practitioner, having assessed the client, informs the latter of what may be needed.
- Feedback. The practitioner gives non-evaluative feedback to the client regarding his behaviour or performance.
- Self-disclosure. The practitioner may offer information about himself or herself and this may help the client understand his situation better.

Other informative interventions are in the form of handouts, visual aids and referrals, which suggest giving the clients details of where they could obtain certain information. In the case of a student for example, a referral type of informative intervention could be, 'the British Lending Library may have a copy of the book you are looking for'.

Informative interventions are perhaps the essence of what helping the client is about. Would it not be great to be able to walk into any new environment and know who's who and what's what? It is of great importance to clients to know what is going on within either their internal or external environment. Such is the need for information, that, it cannot be underestimated. Having said that, the practitioner needs to be aware of when informative interventions can be therapeutic and when they are non-therapeutic. Heron uses the terms 'overdone,' which can be presumed to mean given in over-abundance, and underdone would suggest 'not enough'. Heron (1990) says that when informative intervention is overdone it can interfere with self-directed learning. Similarly when it is underdone, it can disempower people, thus leaving them in ignorance and in the position of becoming victims of oppression.

There are certain criteria which need to be followed for therapeutic interventions and these include:

Criteria for informative interventions

- How much information to give?
- Who to give the information to?
- Whether or not to give information, and whether to let clients find the information for themselves. Heron (1990, p.36) points out, '. . educational reform encourages the move from too much imparting of information by the teacher, to the facilitation of self-directed learning and problem solving in the student'. Whichever side of the fence one happens to be on, one thing to bear in mind is the whole concept of therapeutic intervention. From a personal perspective if giving information will disadvantage the client then it should be withheld. Similarly, if withholding this information will be detrimental to the client, then it should be given. The key issue of 'to give information or not' rests with both practitioner and client. The practitioner needs to be skilled enough to identify the needs of the client. The client on his or her part should, wherever possible, make his or her needs clear to the practitioner.
- Who is the best person to give this information? This does not necessarily have to be the practitioner, it could be any significant other.

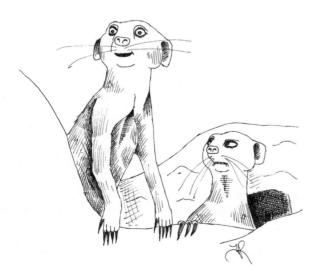

'Is it an eagle? Is it a hawk? No, it's Heron, you're safe'

Confronting interventions

One reason for using confronting interventions is that the clients may not be aware or choose not to be aware of their thoughts, feelings and actions. The practitioner's role is to unveil the mask which actually prevents them from seeing the situation as it truly is. This is not dissimilar to the hypothetical scenario of me being dependent on alcohol and either not realising it or choosing to deny it. The basic interpretation of confronting suggests an element of hostility in behaviour. In fact one of the dictionary definitions of 'confronting' is 'face in hostility or defiance' (*The Pocket Oxford Dictionary of Current English*, 1984, p.150). In a helping scenario, a confronting intervention unmasks or unveils an uncomfortable truth for the client. This act however is carried out with love and the intention to enhance the latter's growth and development.

When to confront?

Here the practitioner finds himself or herself in the position of being a 'Judge', having to decide what the client is aware of or what the client chooses not to be aware of. Similarly the practitioner assumes that it would be in the best interest of the client to become aware of such things. Theoretically it is a sound idea, practically it is one of the most difficult interventions to implement. Heron suggests that if the practitioner has doubts, then deciding upon a contract with the client would help. The contract would basically give the practitioner permission to point out the client's blind spots, without jeopardising the therapeutic relationship.

Effective confronting

Effective confronting is based on practitioners' honesty and sincerity in their intentions. The information which is given to clients about their behaviour needs to be factual and based on evidence and the timing has to be appropriate. If for example you want to confront me about my drinking habit, then you have to make sure you have enough evidence to support the information that you will unmask for me. Do not come to me with, 'well . . . um . . I don't know how to put this. . . .' it will not work. Similarly confronting me long after the event has taken place is a recipe for disaster. Confronting interventions need to take place as soon as it is practical to do so and possibly during or shortly after the event. Heron (1990) says that intervention needs to be on target in content and supportive in manner. It should be truthful but balanced between pussyfooting and the sledge-hammering.

The act of confronting

One of the aims of confronting intervention is to bring to the clients' attention those things which are unknown to them. Heron suggests the following process which needs to be carried out in a clear, uncompromising, non-punitive and non-moralistic manner.

- Identification of the issue of confronting
- Explanation of the practitioner's perception of the clients' blind spot
- Allowing clients time and space to respond to what they have been told about themselves
- Deal with clients' defensive behaviour in a firm and uncompromising way
- Be supportive
- Be direct in questioning

- Deal with clients' avoidance or denial by producing evidence
- Act like a mirror to clients and reflect or mimic what they have said
- Interrupt the clients' pattern of negative behaviour by:
  a drawing attention to something in the immediate environment
  b changing the topic
  c validating what the client is invalidating
  d using diversional activities
- Showing appropriate feelings to clients' behaviour (i.e.) if you are angry then show it. The overall aim of confronting intervention is to increase clients' awareness about issues which they are blind to, in an attempt to promote growth and development. Confronting intervention requires good skills practice to enable its therapeutic value. Having said that, the challenge is such that one can easily slip into a degenerate mode without being aware of it. This may be especially so when dealing with emotion of anger.
- Encouraging self-validation on the part of the client.

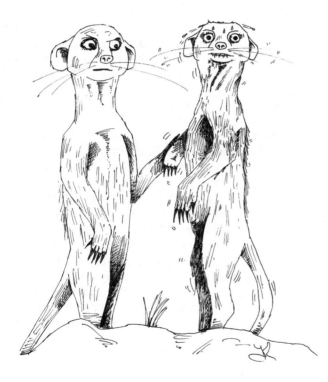

'You said you weren't scared, but how come you're shaking like a leaf?'

1 Reflect on your clinical practice or personal experience and list some of the situations which call for confronting interventions. One such example has already been mentioned (i.e.) someone who is dependent on alcohol and is either unaware of it or denies it.

2 Discuss with a colleague or in groups how a confronting intervention can escalate into a degenerate intervention.

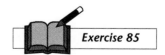

Exercise 85

Cathartic interventions

Catharsis is a Freudian concept which means the release of pent-up emotion. Accordingly therefore, during cathartic interventions the practitioner helps the client to vent painful emotion and undischarged distress that is the cause for his or her disability in the following way:

- Anger is discharged through what Heron calls storming sounds and movements directed without causing harm
- Grief is discharged through tears and sobbing
- Fear is discharged through trembling and shaking
- Embarrassment is discharged through laughter

Catharsis is another one of those interventions which is not to be taken lightly. Heron (1990) states that the process should not start without consent and approval from the client. Catharsis can be seen as a continuum of the release of the various types of tension and these range from 'near the surface – in fresh, spontaneous talk, in ywaning and stretching, and in laughter, to the deeper levels of sobbing, "storming' and trembling,' (Haron, 1990 p.59). The nearer to the surface type of catharsis can be seen as superficial and one could argue that the client is at minimal risk from its application. Clients are much more vulnerable during deeper levels of catharsis.

The 'leading' or 'following' of catharsis

'Leading' in the process of catharsis suggests that the practitioner basically works from his or her hunches, hypotheses and according to his or her own programme. 'Following' means that practitioners work with the cues and clues that they pick up from the clients. In the 'following' role the emphasis is more on what and how clients disclose. The argument here is that the practitioner has to establish a balance between leading and following. Using one at the expense of the other will lead to a degenerate intervention. Heron's view reflects the fact that all leading and no following means indoctrinating the client with the practitioner's agendas, thus ignoring the living presence of the client. In simplistic terms, this would be like total practitioner-centred intervention and would go against the rules of therapeutic intervention. In a similar way, following without any element of leading can lead the practitioner on an aimless journey. Heron suggests a continuous interplay between leading and following as the best way to offer cathartic interventions.

Content versus process

The second dilemma which the practitioner is faced with is the issues of what the client is saying and the way the client is saying it. Again the situation calls for attention being paid to both, one at the expense of the other leads to a degenerative intervention. It is quite possible for the practitioner to be sucked into the client's process of delivery so that valuable elements in the content are missed. Similarly content listening can lead the practitioner on a false trail. An effective practitioner should engage in both the content and the process of the client's catharsis.

Focus of catharsis

Heron identifies three sorts of distress material that the practitioner needs to address and these are the:

- Nature of the distress, which can range from boredom to grief
- Tome of the distress, which can range from the here and now to birth trauma
- Cause of distress, can be interpreted as either intra- or interpersonal or even both. In the case of intrapersonal distress, this is evident in those suffering from depression which is endogenous in nature (the term endogenous means originating from within the person, 'I feel depressed and I am not able to say what is making me feel depressed'. The second type of depression is called reactive because it occurs as a result of a reaction to a loss). Heron suggests physical interference, such as interpersonal interference and nature's interference, such as birth, death and disease as causes of distress.

Heron highlights 40 cathartic interventions with a clear distinction between content and process. Twenty-three of those interventions are content focused and the remaining ones are process focused. All the interventions will not be listed here, but I do however suggest that you refer to Heron's (1990) book, *Helping the Client*. Some of the ways of engaging in a cathartic process with the client are:

Catharsis in practice

1 Asking the client to describe the critical incident which may be one of the contributing factors
2 Asking the client to repeat the words or actions which or she has previously said or done
3 Offering relaxation and light massage
4 Asking the client to offer a literal description of the event
5 Asking the client to relate the story as if it were in the 'here and now,' encouraging the use of the present tense
6 Physically holding or hugging the client (respecting the client's needs)
7 Seeking eye contact
8 Giving the client permission to vent their feelings
9 Inviting the client to relate his or her earliest available memory of events
10 Using psychodrama, this involves asking the client to re-enact the incident
11 Using monodrama, here the client is encouraged to role play the event and he or she plays all the parts

Some of these acts of cathartic intervention are fairly difficult to engage in, competency always rests in practice. Reading about cathartic intervention from these paragraphs or from Heron's work, will contribute to the theoretical know-how, practice, however, remains the key to competency.

Catalytic interventions

A catalytic intervention is one which enables the client to achieve self-directed living. The word 'catalysis' borrowed from the term used in

'It's okay to cry, I did a lot of that when I was a baby'

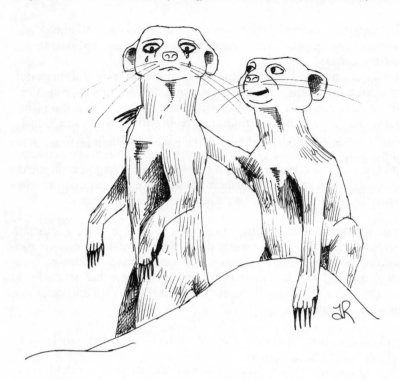

chemistry means helping the client to change so that the latter can live a more independent life. From Heron's (1990) perspective, the purpose of catalytic intervention is to elicit self-discovery, self-directed living, learning and problem solving. The role of the practitioner is to facilitate the process of growth and development on the part of the client. The enabling process includes facilitating the client to:

* Deal with his or her own feelings comfortably
* Reduce the discomfort caused by previous traumas
* Restructure his or her thinking to deal with different sorts of situations
* Develop social and interpersonal skills
* Develop coping mechanisms to deal with crises
* Plan a lifestyle which includes contingency plans in anticipation of change

Catalytic interventions in practice

Heron highlights numerous ways through which catalytic interventions can be facilitated and some of these include:

1   Encouraging the client to make a life map, the content of which could be some of the following:
    * where the client lives
    * the job he or she does
    * education and training
    * personal and professional development

- holidays
- leisure activities
- pleasurable experiences
- physical and psychological traumas
- interpersonal and social relationship

The list can be virtually endless, having said that, the practitioner needs to be skilled enough to deal with any of the issues the client includes in his or her life map.

2   Another version of the life map could be asking the client to focus on the negative aspects or any other aspect of his or her life
3   Exploring past and current events through the process of experimental learning (this concept is discussed in the introduction to this book)
4   Deal with the here and now
5   Deal with the there and then
6   Give free attention
7   Use simple echoing verbal responses
8   Use open and closed questions as appropriate
9   Show empathy
10 Check for understanding
11 Paraphrase the client's sentiments
12 Make use of all the non-verbal cues
13 Work with the client's feelings
14 Offer problem solving structures:
- assessment of situation
- identification of problems
- establishment of objectives (prioritising)
- planning the course of action
- implementation of plan
- reflection, monitoring and evaluation of progress
15 Practitioner's appropriate self-disclosure

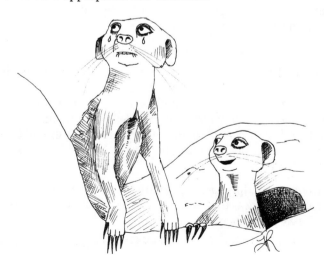

'No, your life map isn't out there, you've got to draw one yourself'

Supportive interventions

Although Heron highlights supportive intervention as a distinct and separate activity, it can be seen as one which in fact filters through all the other interventions. When practitioners are offering prescriptive interventions, they have to be supportive in their approach and the same would apply to informative, confronting, cathartic and catalytic interventions. Having said that, Heron points out that being supportive is a wider concept than the notion of supportive intervention. Being supportive is what Heron calls an attitude of mind that underlies the use of all the other categories of intervention. Some of the specific agendas for a supportive intervention include:

- Being supportive of the person as he or she is
- Being supportive of his or her qualities
- Being supportive of the person's beliefs, values and so on
- Being supportive of what the person does (one can add those behaviours which fall within moral and ethical boundaries)
- Being supportive of the person's creations

Supportive interventions in practice

Supportive interventions can be offered through the practitioner's verbal and non-verbal behaviour. The whole emphasis is focused on the concept of care and love as a therapeutic tool for helping the client. Some of the specific interventions which Heron lists include:

- Expressing the loving feeling
- Expressing care
- Expressing concern
- Validating the client's worth
- Appropriate use of touch
- Sharing and self-disclosing (appropriately)
- Giving free attention
- Encouraging the client
- Giving the client unconditional positive regard
- Accepting the client unconditionally
- Showing warmth

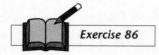

Exercise 86

Understanding the whole concept of six-category interventions in clinical practice can be facilitated through the concept of process recording. A better way of practising the skills of interventions would be to work from a transcribed interview with yourself in the role of the practitioner and a colleague in the role of a client. To this end therefore you should both decide on a scenario, plan and role play the interaction (which could be either audio or video taped).

Work from transcript, identifying and classifying the interventions which are used. Check if they were used appropriately and work out how you could improve on them.

Work out what skills one needs to implement these interventions. I am

'It's good to hug'

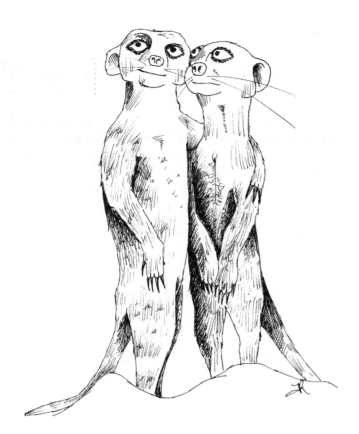

referring here to skills such as, verbal, non-verbal and paralanguage. These would include such factors as listening, attending, responding, paraphrasing, focusing, clarifying, summarising, echoing, etc. There are also those elements which I feel give a human dimension to the art of intervening and these are warmth, acceptance, genuineness and empathy. These issues form the very basis of the concept of helping discussed in Chapter 21.

References

Blake, R. and Mouton, J. (1972). *The Diagnosis and Development Matrix*. Houston, TX: Scientific Methods.

Heron, J. (1990). *Helping The Client: A Creative Practical Guide*. London: Sage.

Mental Health Act (1983). Department of Health and Welsh Office, Code of Practice. London: HMSO.

The Pocket Oxford Dictionary of Current English (1984). 7th edn. Edited by R.E. Allen. Oxford: Clarendon Press.

The concept of helping 21

Objectives

After reading this chapter you should be able to:

1   Explain the notion of helping
2   List some of the helping strategies
3   Describe some of the characteristics of a helper
4   Explain some of the barriers to helping
5   Describe Egan's (1994) model of helping
6   Explain Brammer's (1988) model of helping

Definition of terms

Who is the helper?

Helping means 'Provide (person etc.) with means towards what is needed or sought (helped me with my work; helped me to pay my debts); be of use or service to (person . .); contribute to alleviating (pain or difficulty); . . .' (*The Pocket Oxford Dictionary of Current English*, 1984, p.342). This chapter is concerned with that part of the definition of helping which deals with 'contribute to alleviating pain or difficulty'. The definition of helping could be extended to include the concept of providing the means and support for those who have identified a need for help. Brammer (1988) states that helping is basically a process of enabling people (those in need of help) to grow in the directions that they choose, to solve problems and face crises. From Brammer's perspective therefore, one could argue that helping is an interpersonal activity, during which a person, the helper, facilitates the personal growth and development of another person, the helpee. Who is the helper then? According to Egan (1985), throughout history there has been a firm belief that given the proper conditions, some people are in fact capable of helping others to deal with their personal problems. This belief has now been translated into the roles and functions of the helping professions such as counsellors, psychiatrists, psychologists, social workers, nurses, dentists, general practitioners, lawyers, ministers, teachers and so on. The helper however does not necessarily have to emerge from a health care profession, indeed, a close friend or neighbour can easily slip into that role. The type of helping and the nature of the helper referred to in this chapter is related to health care professionals.

Helping strategies

The numerous ways of helping can range from the helper taking total control of the patient's situation, for instance in dealing with a crisis, to just
being present. Other ways of helping fall into the following categories.

- Giving information and advice implies offering any information
  which the client may need in order to enhance his or her growth
  and development. This is similar to Heron's (1990) concept of informative intervention
- Teaching or educating involves empowering the client with new
  knowledge and skills which will contribute to an independent way
  of life
- Technician, that is, actually doing something or carrying out some
  activities, the result of which leads to alleviating the client's problem
- Changing certain structures in some way. For example if someone is
  physically handicapped, then the internal structure of the house
  may have to be altered to accommodate the client
- Counselling, involves exploring the client's problem with a view to
  providing support
- Being an advocate to the client, safeguarding the interests and welfare of the latter

Portrait of a helper

Rogers (1951) listed some key characteristics which, he argued, are prerequisites to the activities of helping another person. These are:

- Respectful. The implication here is that the helper would see the
  client as a unique being who has dignity, worth and strength
- Genuine. A genuine helper would communicate to the client what is
  felt and thought tactfully
- Attentive. The helper should show the skills of active listening to
  both verbal and non-verbal messages
- Accepting. The helper needs to enable clients to change at their own
  pace, and to acknowledge the clients and their feelings
- Positive. The helper needs to show warmth, caring and should be
  able to reinforce those things that the client does well
- Strong. The helper needs to be able to maintain a separate identity
  from the client and not allow himself or herself to be sucked into
  the client's world
- Knowledgeable. The helper needs to be an expert in his or her field,
  with adequate experience and supervision
- Sensitive. The helper needs to be sensitive to the client's feelings
- Empathic. The helper needs to be able to demonstrate the ability to
  look at the client's world from that particular perspective
- Nonjudgemental. The helper should refrain from making moral
  judgement on the client

- Congruent. The helper needs to be natural, relaxed, trustworthy, dependable and consistent. There is here, a similarity with being genuine which means that the helper needs to be transparent in that his or her outer behaviour should reflect his or her inner self
- Unambiguous. Here again, the helper should not give contradictory messages
- Creative. The helper should view the client as a person who is in the process of becoming and should not cling to the past
- Secure. The helper needs to allow the client to remain separate and unique, showing respect for the client's needs and emotions
- The helper needs to feel safe as the client moves closer, without feeling the need to exploit the latter

It is generally believed that in order to be a helper, one needs to:

1   Be committed to one's own growth and development
2   Model the behaviour one hopes to help others to achieve
3   Know how to help oneself
4   Show respect to oneself
5   Be a good learner and translator, for instance, be able to recognise verbal and non-verbal cues
6   Be non-defensive
7   Be spontaneous
8   Care for the interest of one's client
9   Be able to make use of appropriate self-disclosure
10 Be able to explore one's own behaviour, recognising and accepting who one is

It can be concluded from this list that the main requirements of being a helper are focused around issues of:

- self-awareness
- reflection
- knowledge, skills and
- attitudes

Barriers to helping

There are obviously numerous barriers to the helping relationship between the practitioner and the client. For the sake of clarity, these will be explored from three perspectives, which are the practitioner, the client and the environment.

The practitioner as a barrier to the helping process

Although the implication is that anyone who occupies the role of helper, should have the client's interest at heart, nevertheless this is not always the case. In every professional arena, there are what would be seen as good and poor (bad) workers and the health care situation is no exception. Those who are bad can be grouped under two categories and these are:

- bad through intention
- bad through ignorance (like in lack of skills)

These are what Heron (1990) called perverted and degenerate interventions respectively (these concepts were discussed in Chapter 20). Barriers to helping therefore, can be due to both a perverted and a degenerate practitioner. The remedy in the case of the former can only be through dismissal and of the latter through education. Other factors which can interfere (negatively) with the helping process include:

- The practitioner's attitude, values and beliefs
- The practitioner's motivation (lack of commitment for personal growth)
- The practitioner's non-acceptance of the client
- The practitioner's over-involvement with the client (like in sexual intimacy)
- The practitioner's dependency on the client (as exemplified by Berne's concept of symbiosis, see Chapter 13)
- The practitioner's lack of respect for the client and for self
- The practitioner's false front (like in putting up a façade)
- The practitioner's lack of communication skills (for instance being unable to listen, attend and respond)
- The practitioner's lack of sensitivity
- The practitioner's judgmental attitude
- The practitioner's personal problems
- The practitioner's defensiveness
- The practitioner's inappropriate self-disclosure
- The practitioner's inability to work with difficult emotions
- The practitioner's expectation (for example expecting too much from the client)
- The practitioner's lack of self-awareness

The client as a barrier to the helping process

Although it is difficult to conceptualise that the client, who is in need of help, can in fact be a barrier to the helping process, nevertheless it is not uncommon to observe such a dynamic. There are in fact numerous factors which can lead the client to being a hindrance to the process of helping and some of these are:

- The client's non-compliance
- The client's lack of motivation and interest
- The client's lack of insight into the severity of the problems
- The client's lack of respect for self and others
- The client's lack of disclosure
- The client's attitude, values and beliefs
- The client's defensiveness
- The client's learned helplessness
- The client's passive role
- The client's preference for the sick role
- The client's expectation of the practitioner's role (they may expect the practitioner to sort the problem out)

- The client's perception of problem (they may consider it unsolvable and hopeless)
- The client's lack of self-awareness (they may be unaware of their own strengths)

The environment as a barrier to the helping process

Environment is taken to include both the psychological and the physical. The psychological environment would include such factors as:

- The client's feeling that they are not safe or secure
- The client's perception of lack of warmth and caring on the part of the practitioner
- The client's lack of a sense of comfort with the practitioner

From a physical perspective, barriers would include:

- The physical structure of the room
- The positioning of the practitioner (that is, posture and proximity)
- Noise
- Lack of privacy
- Too warm, too cold or lack of ventilation
- Uncomfortable chairs
- Interruptions (like telephone calls or a knock on the door)
- Distractions inside or outside the room

Helping models

There are numerous approaches to helping, for example, Rogers' concept of client-centred therapy focuses on viewing the client's problem from his or her perspective; Ellis's (1973) concept of rational emotive therapy on the other hand, emphasises changing the client's irrational ways of thinking into rational thinking; Perls' (1973) focus was on the whole person in the 'here and now' scenario. The approaches which are explored in this chapter are those of Egan (1975) and Brammer (1988).

Egan's model of helping

Egan first formulated the concept of *The Skilled Helper* in 1975, with the latest revision made in 1994. The model is described as a problem-management approach to helping, and it is basically structured around three stages. These stages are:

1   Reviewing the current scenario. The principle here is to help the client identify, explore, and clarify their problem situations and unused opportunities.
2   Developing the preferred scenarios. The principle here is to help the client identify where they want to go and what they want to do with their problem situations and opportunities.
3   Getting there. The principle here is to help the client formulate some action plan to achieve what they want.

An example of this model is to suppose that I am uncomfortable and unhappy with my current situation in Leeds and I want to get out. Both my helper and I establish my best option, that is, to be in London and then set to work on finding the most feasible way of getting there. There are however numerous steps both helper and client have to go through in order for the client to reach their objective and these are discussed below.

This stage sees the primary goal as the identification of the problems the client is faced with. This therefore is where it all starts, the helper and the client embark on a journey of discovering what lies ahead of them. Egan highlights three steps which form the basis of the first stage, these are steps:

Stage I   Reviewing problem situations and unused opportunities

A   Helping the clients to tell and clarify their stories
B   Identifying and challenging blind spots
C   Searching for leverage

How does one help clients to tell their stories? This is the time to resource all those communication skills which have been discussed previously. So as a way of reflecting, have a go at Exercise 87.

Helping clients to tell their stories

Make a list of some of the communication skills you will use to enable the clients to describe their situations. This activity is best carried out on an individual basis initially, then discuss your findings with your colleagues or group.

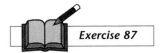

Exercise 87

As Egan said, some clients may be quite verbal whilst others may be practically mute. Opening up to a complete stranger is not something which comes naturally to anyone. There are key factors which can contribute to either facilitating or hindering this process. First and foremost, clients need to feel safe, secure, comfortable and trusting, before they can 'tell their stories'. It goes without saying therefore that as a professional caregiver, one needs to work on establishing or creating a psychological and physical environment which will enhance the clients' disclosure. This is described as 'relationship building', and Egan (1985, p.37) had the following to say about it. 'Relationship building is also central to the entire process. A good working relationship is one that contributes to productive outcomes in the counselling sessions.' Some of the issues which Rogers identified as characteristics of a helper come into play here. These include:

- Respect for the clients
- Genuine, congruency, trusting, sincere and honest
- Good listening, attending and responding skills (these would include questioning skills)
- Accepting
- Empathic understanding
- Being non-judgmental

The implication here is that clients may be so engrossed into their problems that they do not have an objective view of the whole situation. The

Identifying and challenging blind spots

role of the helper in this instance is to 'identify blind spots and develop new, more useful perspectives on both problem situations and unused opportunities' (Egan, 1994, p.26). The whole purpose of challenging the clients' blind spots is to help them see themselves and everything around them in a more creative way. This is reflected in Heron's (1990) concept of confronting intervention.

Searching for leverage

This step revolves round the issues of screening, focusing and clarifying. Egan argues that because helping is a financially and psychologically expensive proposition, some sort of screening is needed. Screening is taken to mean establishing:

1   whether the problem is worth the time and effort for its manage-ment
2   the number of problems identified
3   the complexity of the problems
4   the order of priority to deal with the problems

The need for screening is important in that it establishes a certain boundary and offers a structure to work from. Take the last point, 'establish the order of priority,' it may well be that the resolution of the one problem may help to solve the remaining problems. Similarly if in an attempt to deal with one problem, numerous other problems were to emerge, then serious consideration has to be given to whether to deal with the problem or not.

Stage II   Developing the preferred scenario

Helping the client to develop the preferred scenario has a further three steps:

A   Developing what the client sees as the preferred scenario possibilities
B   Translating these possibilities into viable objectives
C   Commitment to the change

Developing preferred scenario possibilities

Egan (1994, pp.30–31) states that 'the principle function in developing the preferred scenario possibilities is to help clients develop a range of avenues for a better future'. Clients are helped with such questions as, 'What do I really want? What would my life look like if it looked better?. . . . What would this problem situation look like if managed? What would be in place that is not now in place? What would this opportunity look like if it were developed? What would exist that does not exist at this moment?' Both the helper and client work on what is realistic for the client to achieve.

Translating possibilities into viable goals

The focus of translating possibilities into viable objectives is on finding out what clients really want against what is realistic to achieve. The clients' possibilities need to be workable and within what is available. If clients are setting unrealistic objectives, then it is up to the helper to ensure that all possibilities have been explored. Egan (1985, p.45) argues, 'often helpers need to challenge clients to make vague goals more specific'.

Commitment to a programme of constructive change

The focus of this stage is to help clients to identify the incentives that will encourage them to pursue their goals. How committed are the clients to want to get better? And how much will clients do for themselves to achieve their goals? What price are they prepared to pay? Personal experience suggests that some clients will contract to help themselves but then found out that they just can't do it. Some may prefer to stay in their present situation. All these need to be clarified and only then both helper and client may be able to move forward.

The journey thus far has meant establishing what the current state of affairs are, for example where the clients want to go. This stage deals with how to get where the clients want to go. Here too there are three steps and these are:

Stage III   Determining how to get there

A   Brainstorming strategies for action
B   Choosing the best strategies
C   Turning strategies into plan

The helper works with the client to brainstorm ways of achieving the goals. The presumption here is that there is more than one way of achieving what one wants. It would therefore seem pointless to work with the first one that comes to mind. Other ways may prove to be more economical in many ways. Furthermore if the chosen strategy proves too difficult, clients can always opt for the second avenue.

Brainstorming strategies for action

The focus here is to help clients to select the particular strategies which would be best suited for the:

Choosing the best strategies

*   environment
*   resources
*   client's capability
*   client's needs

The aim of this particular step is to consider every possibility from a realistic perspective. Egan (1994) states that realism is important because it is pointless to choose strategies that can lead only to failure. Sometimes clients will choose something more challenging, this is okay provided this challenge is not going to turn into a threat. Similarly one could say that the easiest strategies may not always the best option.

Plans are formulated according to their place in the hierarchy of priorities. These plans are detailed to the point that clients are quite clear as to what they are suppose to do and by which time they are to achieve their goals. Having said that, clients need to be helped to prepare themselves for implementing the plans. They also need to be warned of the difficulties they may encounter during the implementation of these plans. If no warning is given in terms of possible obstacles, clients may be under the illusion that things from here on in would run smoothly. Egan calls this, 'to be forewarned is to be forearmed'. If I know the danger which lies ahead of me I can prepare myself. If not this will come as a shock to me.

Turning strategies into a plan

Egan stresses the point that each of the steps need to be evaluated as an ongoing process and evaluation should not be seen as an appendage which is attached to the end of the helping process.

Evaluation

Brammer's (1988) model of helping

Brammer's (1988) model of helping emphasises two major phases and these are:

1 Building relationships phase. This is made up of four stages:
   - entry
   - clarification
   - structure
   - relationship
2 Facilitating positive action phase. This phase also is made up of four stages:
   - exploration
   - consolidation
   - planning
   - termination

Preparing and entering into the relationship

This is the stage when the helper and the client meet. Brammer sees the goals here as:

- Opening the interview with the minimal of resistance
- Laying the groundwork for trust
- Enabling the client to state his or her request for help clearly and comfortably

The main foci of this stage are for both helpers and clients to deal with:

- Readiness. The key issue is seen as the need on the part of the helper to establish, define and reflect on what it is that the client wants in this stage of the relationship
- Resistance. Although it is the clients themselves who come for help, there are times when they show resistance in the helping process. This may be due to the fact that they are afraid of confronting and dealing with their own feelings. Brammer (1988) identifies other issues such as:

  1 Receiving help can be difficult
  2 Commitment to change can be difficult
  3 Being a helpee can be a threat to one's esteem, integrity, and sense of independence
  4 Trusting strangers is not a natural phenomenon
  5 One can so easily be blind to one's own problem
  6 Perception of one's problem can be too overwhelming to share with the helper
  7 Culture may inhibit one's search for help.

- Environment (setting). The implication is that the environment does contribute to the sense of comfort and security of clients. This would include all those factors, such as proxemics and gaze, which have been discussed earlier

- Opening of the interview. This, in a way, can be seen as breaking the ice

I shall leave this, opening of the interview, for you to work out in Exercise 88.

Assuming that this is the first time you have met your client, make a list of the different opening statements you could use to initiate your client into telling his or her story. Make sure none of your opening statements sound too threatening, too direct or are likely to make your client feel uncomfortable.

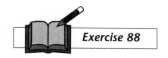

Exercise 88

It may also be useful to work out what you feel the possible answers may be. Explore whether each response gives you what you want to know.

Clarification

The whole issue of clarification is to make sure as a helper one understands what the client's problems are about. This is dealt with in Chapter 17 under the heading of 'Listening, attending and responding'. Investigate questioning, focusing, reflecting, echoing and so on. Brammer states that this clarification stage should also provide the helper with such information as, where to go for the remaining stages and what to do next. The term treatment planning is applied in formal helping situations. Clarification will also lead the helper to distinguish who owns the problem. The problem may be the client's or any significant others. Some clients may come for help, when the problem in fact belongs to someone else. The reverse can also apply, clients may come for help on behalf of another member of the family, when it is they themselves who have the problems.

Structure

This stage focuses on the terms and conditions of the working relationship. Brammer (1988), offers a list of questions, which must be answered by both the client and the helper in order to establish whether the relationship can proceed. As a helper you should ask yourself questions such as

- Can, or better still, do I want to work with this patient?
- Similarly the client should ask himself or herself the same question
- Can I trust him or her?
- Will I have control of my commitment and involvement?

The structure stage of the helping process is said to include such issues as formulating contracts and role responsibilities.

Relationship

According to Brammer, by the time the fourth stage is reached, the helper–client relationship should be firmly established, where trust and openness are strengthened. Brammer sees silence as a very important factor at this stage.

Exploration

By the time this level is reached, the helper will have a clear idea of what the problems are and will take on a more active and assertive role. Exploration is focused on the changes and the strategies that need to be employed in order to get the patient where he or she wants to be. Brammer highlights eight key points which he believes are important in achieving these changes. These are:

1   Maintaining and enhancing the relationship
2   Examining and dealing with resistance on the part of both the client and the helper
3   Encouraging the client to explore his or her problems or feelings further in an attempt to enhance self-awareness
4   Encouraging the client to clarify and further specify his or her goals
5   Collecting data which would help the client
6   Deciding whether to continue or terminate the relationship
7   Teaching the client skills which he or she will need to solve the problems
8   Initiating homework activities, which will help the client to reach his or her goals

This stage may also involve the concept of transference and countertransference. Transference is said to take place when the client projects feelings, which he or she once felt toward someone close, onto the helper. 'Helpees may see their fathers symbolically in the helper, who now has a position of some authority and power, and they may respond to the helper in the same way they responded to their fathers in earlier years' (Brammer, 1988, p.61). Countertransference on the other hand is a similar phenomenon to transference except that it is the helper who projects his or her feelings onto the client as a direct response to the latter's transference.

Consolidation

The function at this stage is to embark on the task of settling on alternative choices of practising the new skills. This is also the time when the client needs to act instead of talking. The main focus here is to clarify feelings, settle for alternative actions and practice new skills.

Planning

This stage sees the planning of the termination of the client–helper relationship. The client needs to prepare to live as independent a life as possible. This is like a 'weaning' process in preparation for the termination stage.

Termination

This stage may involve a reflection and summary of the whole process. The termination stage can be tailored to suit both client and helper, the focus however should be on leaving the client with the feeling that termination does not necessarily mean that the door is closed, so they cannot come back again. Clients need to be made aware that support still exists even after the helping process. This can be seen as leaving the door open to give the client a sense of security that he or she can always come back for support.

One could argue that both Egan and Brammer have offered similar views regarding the concept of helping. These can be summarised as

Assessment of problems
Identification of problems
Selecting priorities
Planning of the actual process of helping
Implementation of the actual process of helping and
Evaluation of both the helping process itself and its effect on the client

The dynamics of the helping process rest with initiation maintenance and termination of the relationship between professional caregiver and client. Underpinning the whole process of helping are the theoretical knowledge and practical skills and attitude, which have as their foundation the element of self-awareness. Self-awareness in turn can be enhanced by self-reflection. Reflection forms the basis of Chapter 22.

References

Brammer, L.M. (1988). *The Helping Relationship; Process and Skills*. London: Allyn and Bacon.

Egan, G. (1977). *The Skilled Helper*. Monterey, CA: Brooks/Cole.

Egan, G. (1985). *The Skilled Helper: A Systematic Approach To Effective Helping*. Pacific Grove, CA: Brooks/Cole.

Egan, G. (1994). *The Skilled Helper: A Systematic Approach To Effective Helping*. Pacific Grove, CA: Brooks/Cole.

Ellis, A. (1973). *Humanistic Psychotherapy: The Rational-Emotive Approach*. New York: McGraw-Hill.

Heron, J. (1990). *Helping The Client: A Creative Practical Guide*. London: Sage.

The Pocket Oxford Dictionary of Current English (1984). 7th edn. Edited by R.E. Allen. Oxford: Clarendon Press.

Perls, F.S. (1973). *The Gestalt Approach*. Palo Alto, CA: Science and Behaviour Books. (Paperback edition, New York: Bantam, 1976).

Rogers, C.R. (1951). *Client Centred Therapy*. London: Constable.

Reflection and conclusion 22

Objective

After reading this chapter you should be able to recognise and appreciate that the standard of care delivery rests with effectiveness of communication and that self-awareness is the fulcrum of any therapeutic relationship.

Reflection in this context is taken to mean, the act of looking back and critically analysing the issues which have emerged during the course of the discussions in previous chapters. With this in mind, the intention is to link the concept of self-awareness with care delivery. An attempt is made here at explaining how by being self-aware one is able to enhance care delivery. The starting point is with Berne's (1961) concept of transactional analysis.

Self-awareness transactional analysis and care delivery

Awareness of one's ego states

Transactional analysis offers people opportunities to discover their true self and to change if they so wish. It needs to be stressed that when people's internal dynamics are made more visible to them, communication can be much more effective. As a carer, one's responsibility is to ensure that complementary transactions are initiated and sustained throughout a helper–client interaction. The helper also needs to avoid engaging in crossed and ulterior transactions. When these are encountered, the helper's responsibility is to try to channel the transactions into complementary ones. Crossed and ulterior transactions can only lead to negative outcomes and hence become non-therapeutic interventions. Having said that, this does not mean that the helper has to be in total agreement with the client. Any differences of opinion can be dealt with on an amicable basis, and this is the very reason for learning the skills of interpersonal communication. Clients are, in most cases, at a disadvantage in that they are in need of care in one form or another, helpers, on the other hand, are in the privileged position of being the caregivers. They are perceived as authority figures by virtue of their status, knowledge and skill. It goes without saying therefore that if there is any changing of behaviour to be done, it has to come from the helpers first. Only when helpers have established that the need to change rests with the clients, can the latter be confronted in a supportive manner.

Since ego states are the driving forces of behaviour, one needs to be aware of the nature of these forces. This is not dissimilar to being aware of gear changes when driving a car. It would not do to drive at 50 miles per hour in first gear, similarly it would be a bad idea to use one's critical parent ego state when interacting with a client who has a negative self-concept. Being familiar with one's ego states will enable the helper to balance out his or her feelings and thinking and to respond in a manner which will enhance therapeutic communication.

By its very definition, transactional analysis implies looking closely at how transactions between two or more people are formed. Structural analysis on the other hand, offers an insight into the origin of each statement that the interactants make. Equipped with this information, the helper should be able to monitor his or her behaviour during any interaction. An awareness that crossed transactions can only lead to negative outcome and bad feelings would motivate one towards trying to convert these into complementary transactions especially in a helper role. As a health care professional, one would use such skills as listening, attending with the appropriate responses and checking for understanding. The underpinning philosophy would be 'if I am not getting the response that I need, I have to be aware of what I am doing, in turn, I will discover why I am not getting the desired response'. This is not dissimilar to trying to fit a square peg in a round hole. If the medium or the content of my communication is incompatible, I may have to alter them so that my message is received by the appropriate ego state of the client, who in turn responds from an ego state which I desire. For example as a helper if I communicate with a client from my critical parent ego state when I should have been communicating from my nurturing parent ego state, the resulting intervention would be perceived by the client as non-therapeutic. From this perspective, self-awareness holds the key to enhancing a client's growth, development and independence.

Life-positions and their influences on care delivery

From Inhelder and Piaget's (1958) and Tolman's (1958) points of view, behaviour can be understood by analysing one's schema of things or of events. The implication is that people would behave according to how they view the world around them. From a cognitive perspective, thought and perception are two of the most influential factors in the way people respond to their environment. If an individual occupies the life-position of 'I'm OK and you're OK,' he or she is functioning from a healthy state of mind. If, on the other hand, one occupies the three other life-positions, 'I'm OK – you're not OK,' 'I'm not OK – you're OK,' and 'I'm not OK – you're not OK,' the resulting thoughts and beliefs could be described as irrational. This could have serious implications if helpers are unaware of their own true thoughts. In the first two instances, carers would come across as aggressive (I'm OK – you're not OK) and submissive (I'm not OK – you're OK). An aggressive helper is an unapproachable person and similarly a submissive helper becomes degenerate due to a lack of skill.

Awareness of one's thoughts can enhance care delivery especially if the helper is egocentric. Being egocentric would suggest that the carer is unable to see it from the client's perspective. This means the former would be unable to empathise with clients.

Every health care professional needs to be aware that each individual has different moral principles and reasoning. If as a carer, I condemn the very idea of abortion or of euthanasia, I need to recognise that these are my beliefs and that others may feel differently. I should therefore learn to accept others as individuals with their own needs and feelings. What is right and proper for one is not necessarily the same for others. The nature of the caring professions is such that one will undoubtedly have to help people from different walks of life, for example some may be petty criminals whilst others may be murderers. If one is aware of one's values, beliefs and moral principles, then one will be in a better position to be able to do something about these. This could be anything from asking someone else to care for that person, to actively accepting the latter for who he or she is rather than for what he or she has done. Rogers would call this unconditional acceptance, which in many ways is a very difficult thing to do.

Self-awareness of one's perceptions and their influences on helping behaviour

As Hastorft *et al.*'s (1970) views reflect, the world is not merely revealed to people, instead, they play active roles in creating their own experiences. This implies that what one sees is one's own creation and not necessarily what is actually in view. It is 'reality' as the perceiver experiences it. A person who has visual hallucinations may say that he or she has seen Jesus. This is not dissimilar to the idea that 12 plus 1 is 1. For example in a 12-hour clock 12 plus 1 is 1. From this perspective, one can only assume that reality can only exist in the mind of each individual and what the individual perceives is his or her true experience at any particular time. Leeper's (1935) finding suggests that the first encounter may be a lasting experience or it may even be the only experience one is ready to take on board. The implication may well be that if a client displays aggressive behaviour on the first encounter, this may become a fixed schema the helper chooses to accept. Any non-aggressive behaviour is most likely going to be ignored. The perceived image can be nothing but distorted. The categorisational feature of perception would come into play and the helper will be biased in his/her approach to the client. An awareness of the fact that if I wear a pair of glasses with red lenses, the colour that I see can only be red, should in fact enable me to recognise and acknowledge that my internal frame of reference will directly influence the way I perceive my clients. Similarly if a helper was to ascribe a label to a client, the latter can only be seen through that label and no other attributes may be picked up.

Humanistic influence and the concept of care

It could be argued that the humanistic approach to understanding human behaviour is one of the very few perspectives which focuses on the individual's conscious awareness. The belief that each individual is unique in his or her own right, provides the avenue for the helper to recognise and accept that clients retain their individuality regardless of the roles they find themselves in. Such individuality emphasises an awareness of one's own experience, being the creator of one's destiny, being able to choose freely and being responsible for one's own existence. The inner goodness of each individual will emerge provided he/she is guided and helped to grow and develop. One of the reasons the individual shows cruel or sadistic behaviour is that his or her needs may be frustrated. This is not difficult to understand in the sense that if any one of us is to be prevented from satisfying what we feel our needs or goals to be, we would show our displeasure in one way or another. The individual is also seen as an integrated whole. If for example my little toe hurts then the whole of 'me' suffers and not just my toe. There is not any one part of the body which functions independently. A dynamic exists between the whole of the body and the whole of the soul. The wants and the needs belong to the whole person and not to his or her individual parts. Recognition of these in oneself should enable the helper to realise these in others. As far as human needs are concerned, both client and helper share a set of universal basic needs which have to be satisfied in an hierarchical order. Having said that, the priority of satisfaction is not necessarily the same for everyone and each has his or her own individual target for self-actualisation. This leads one to believe that people should be left to function at their own pace towards their own personal goals.

Rogers (1951) introduced the idea of phenomenal field into the concept of caring to suggest that the helper considers the sum total of the client's experience. Similarly if one wants to know how the client is feeling, then one has to ask the client, because the latter is better placed than anyone else to be able to tell it as it really feels. The interplay between a person's 'figure and ground' points to the fact that, what is unconscious can become conscious and vice versa. It is just a question of what one is aware of at any one particular time.

Whose vantage point is it anyway?

Awareness of the fact that an individual will do almost anything to gain positive regard and acceptance should enable the helper to protect the vulnerability of clients. Clients should be unconditionally valued. Similarly the helper's internal responses should be congruent with his/her external behaviour. Roughly translated this means that I should be transparent in that I should behave how I think and feel. Perhaps one should pause and critically analyse this issue. To truly behave how one thinks and feels may not necessarily lead to therapeutic interventions. What if I feel a dislike towards my students, what purpose would it serve for me to disclose this information? In fact at best this could be seen as a degenerate intervention for my lack of skills and at worst it would be perceived as perverted because I would have benefited from having vented this feeling. What should one do then? This is one of those 'Catch 22' situations, perhaps the only way out would be to assess the state of the client and establish whether or not the latter would gain from such a disclosure. The helper however should not lose sight of what he/she truly thinks and how he/she truly feels. Recognising and acknowledging those emotions which one

Unconditional positive regards and helping

finds difficult to deal with in oneself is a recipe for good interpersonal communication. The same would apply to recognising and acknowledging those emotions one finds difficult to deal with in others.

Awareness of one's needs for satisfaction and security

It could be argued from Sullivan's (1953) perspective that an individual is driven by the need for satisfaction and security. The need for satisfaction is achieved by a state of euphoria in ridding oneself of tension. This could be linked with the very reason for one's existence, that is, one lives for the search of pleasure. Satisfying the need for security is achieved by ridding oneself of anxiety. A parallel could be drawn here between the mother–infant relationship and the helper–client relationship. According to Sullivan, an anxious mother would unknowingly instil anxiety in the infant. It could be argued that an anxious helper too will instil anxiety in the client. An awareness of one's anxious state would allow the helper an opportunity to reflect on and deal with his/her own intrapersonal dynamics. There is no implication here to suggest that all helpers instil anxiety in clients. Having said that those who are anxious will in fact generate clients' anxiety by their very behaviour. This is based on the principle that a helper who is anxious will not be perceived as confident by the client. The latter may then feel insecure and this in turn may generate anxiety.

Selective inattention, focal awareness and care delivery

It is human nature for an individual to have a tendency not to notice certain things in his/her life, especially if this involves tension. Outside his or her roles, the helper is a human being. This therefore means that the helper too has moments of selective inattention. As a lecturer, I may not pay attention to a so-called 'difficult' student. Similarly a helper may not pay attention to an 'unpopular' client. Focal awareness means that one functions from one's own hidden agendas, for example I may choose to see or hear what I want to see or hear, rather than how it really is. The tri-components of one's attitude offer an insight into the dynamics between internal response and external behaviour. Lack of awareness of these dynamics will create a state of unconscious incompetence.

Learning and care delivery

Behavioural and social learning theories emphasise the significance of environmental influences on the organism. Watson's principles of associative learning could make a patient's experience pleasant or unpleasant depending on the environment health care professionals provide. This type of learning is mostly unconscious and reflexive. Changes in one's behaviour are mostly insidious and unknown until displayed by external behaviour. Lack of awareness could lead to continuous reinforcement of undesired behaviour. For example my internal response could lead me to feel uncomfortable in my interaction with you and in turn an aversion may be created. Hence I take a dislike to you and avoid your presence as much as possible. Similarly from an operant point of view, if I feel rewarded by your presence, I may end up liking you more. This notion is reflected in Stockwell's concept of the 'unpopular patient'.

To what extent does one copy or imitate the behaviour of others? One could argue that this is much more than could be imagined. Here also there is an element of unconscious internal dynamism. It goes on all the time except one may not be aware of it. A typical example would be 'how one's accent changes as one moves to a different place in the country'. Transferring this concept to health care settings, one could easily pick up other people's ways of working. Excellent role models would contribute to a high standard of care delivery. The reverse would also be true in that viruses would be spread from those negative role models and the whole of the environment would be contaminated to such an extent that this particular way of working would become the norm. Such is the impact of influence that the practitioner is rendered unconsciously incompetent. One's own self-awareness is the only virus killer one has at one's disposal.

Power, control and self-awareness

Zimbardo's (1992) concept of deindividuation suggests that one of the ways of taking power and control from an individual is to remove that person's identity, as was obvious in his prison experiment. Those students who put on prisoners' clothes lost their own identities and those who put on their guards' uniforms underwent a change of attitude. Both groups of people were seen to exhibit two sets of behaviour. Those civilians who previously would have been self dependent became helpless prisoners and those of a humanistic nature became cruel and sadistic guards. One of the factors that appeared to have contributed to the change in behaviour was the issue of control. One group had no control whilst the other group had total control. A parallel can be drawn in some health care settings between patients and helpers' roles. Some patients will consciously or unconsciously give control to their helpers. Control or perceived control is the main issue in the concept of learned helplessness. One can unconsciously create learned helplessness in patients in a variety of ways and these include:

- Withholding information (consciously or unconsciously)
- Creating dependency by dictating care rather than facilitating its process
- Planning patients' care without involving them
- Taking the role of a 'doer', that is offering unsolicited help

One can actually guard against the inducement of learned helplessness in patients by exploring one's own personal philosophy regarding people and the concept of caring. I could for example ask myself the following questions.

Do I tell the patients what they want to know or
Do I tell them what I want them to hear?
Do I do things for patients because they cannot do it for themselves or
Because I am in a rush and other jobs need to be done?
Do I consult patients about their needs or
Do I offer help based on what I feel they need?

The answers to these types of question will dictate the kind of carer/helper one is. An awareness of these should in fact motivate one into action.

Leadership styles and care delivery

The three styles of leadership, authoritarian, democratic and laissez-faire, identified by Lewin *et al.* (1939), have implications for the way one cares for patients. Perhaps it would be true to say that authoritarian leaders in terms of task-oriented groups emerge as leaders of leaders. This suggests that the group will be highly productive but at the expense of suffering from low morale. In health care settings, patients would enjoy knowing that they are in safe, but unfortunately, cold hands. Democratic leaders on the other hand are described as person oriented and seem to be more concerned with satisfying the needs of their members but at the expense of lengthy decision-making processes. Laissez-faire leaders do not really want to be leaders and subordinates feel an element of insecurity in the lack of guidance and direction. This will not be reassuring for patients. As a carer one needs to assess the needs of patients in the context of their situation and offer the style of leadership which is warranted.

A formula for care

Self-awareness means being in touch with one's thoughts, feelings and actions. This therefore suggests being consciously aware of one's own existence. As a helper recognising and accepting my Values, Idiosyncrasies, Attitudes, Strengths, Weaknesses, Assumptions and Beliefs as unique to me, will lead me to recognise and accept your V.I.A.S.W.A.B. as unique to you. When I care for you, I need to look at your situation from your vantage point and this will enable me to have a better understanding of your problem. If I look at your situation from my perspective, the picture that I see will be a blur because my eyes will not be in focus. Caring therefore is about seeing and feeling it from the client's own frame of reference and the ability to do so rests with the concept of self-awareness.

References

Berne, E. (1961). *Transactional Analysis in Psychotherapy. The Classic Handbook to its Principles*. New York: Grove Press.

Hastorft, H.A., Schneider, D.J. and Ppolefka, J. (1970). *Person Perception*. Reading, MA: Addison-Wesley.

Inhelder, B. and Piaget, J. (1958). *The Growth of Logical Thinking from Childhood to Adolescence*. New York: Basic Books. London: Routledge and Kegan Paul.

Leeper, R. (1935). 'The role of motivation in learning. A study of the phenomenon of differential motivation control of the utilisation of habits.' *Journal of Genetic Psychology*, 46, 3–40.

Lewin, K., Lippitt, R. and White, R. (1939). 'Patterns of aggressive behaviour in experimentally created "social climates."' *Journal of Social Psychology*, 10, 271–299.

Rogers, C.R. (1951). *Client Centred Therapy*. London: Constable.

Sullivan, H.S. (1953). *The Interpersonal Theory of Psychiatry*. New York: Norton.

Tolman, E.C. (1958). *Essays in Motivation and Learning*. Berkeley, CA: University of California Press.

Zimbardo, P. (1992). *Psychology of Life*. New York: Harper Collins.

Index

Headings are arranged in word-by-word alphabetical order. Page references in *italics* denote figures and tables